BEATING ENDO

BEATING ENDO

How to Reclaim Your Life

from Endometriosis

Iris Kerin Orbuch, MD

Amy Stein, DPT

HARPER WAVE

An Imprint of HarperCollinsPublishers

BEATING ENDO. Copyright © 2019 by Iris Kerin Orbuch and Amy Stein. All rights reserved. Printed in the United States of America. No part of this book may be used or reproduced in any manner whatsoever without written permission except in the case of brief quotations embodied in critical articles and reviews. For information, address HarperCollins Publishers, 195 Broadway, New York, NY 10007.

HarperCollins books may be purchased for educational, business, or sales promotional use. For information, please email the Special Markets Department at SPsales@harpercollins.com.

FIRST EDITION

Designed by William Ruoto

Illustrations courtesy of Marie Dauenheimer

Photos courtesy of Richard Hutchings

Library of Congress Cataloging-in-Publication Data has been applied for.

ISBN 978-0-06-286183-2

19 20 21 22 23 LSC 10 9 8 7 6 5 4 3 2 1

To the one-tenth of all women on earth who are estimated to have endometriosis, and to those among them who have been our patients

CONTENTS

FOREWORD

BOJANA NOVAKOVIC

I had pelvic pain for more than two decades—and didn't know why. As a teenager, I was told it was normal for girls to have painful periods; when I became sexually active, I was told it was normal for sex to hurt. A laparoscopy in 2005 came up negative for endometriosis; I now know the surgeon most likely did not know what she was looking for. Because endo had been ruled out as a cause, I was told the pain was in my head, or that sex hurt because I was uptight and anxious. Everyone I turned to pointed the finger back at me, so I started looking inward. My anxiety increased; the more pain there was, the more I worried that I was doing something wrong. This cycle of confusion, pain, and discomfort wreaked havoc on my mind, body, and central nervous system for fifteen years.

I'm no scientist, but I can say with complete confidence: There is nothing normal about knife-stabbing pain during your period, nausea with bowel movement during your period, burning, itching, tingling pain sporadically throughout your cycle—and definitely nothing normal about pain during intercourse. Even though women go through the painful act of childbirth, PAIN IS NOT SYNONYMOUS WITH BEING FEMALE. Possessing female reproductive organs doesn't condemn you to eternal pain. We all know that life hurts. We all struggle. But pelvic pain is not a metaphor for life. It's a real ailment with causes and conditions—and it can be treated.

My cause was endometriosis, but it lasted so long that I grew used to its symptoms and figured out how to "put up" with them. In November 2017, I started to experience severe lethargy and intestinal pain that six months of testing finally identified as SIBO—small intestinal bacterial overgrowth—which, like endo, is an inflammatory condition. By that time, I was also seeing a physical therapist specializing in pelvic pain during sex. Both the GI doctor and the physical therapist suggested I see Dr. Orbuch, proposing that the symptoms I was experiencing could be from long-standing endometriosis.

It's difficult for an intelligent, well-read, independent woman like myself to contemplate that what a medical expert had once assured her was *not* the cause of her lifelong pain might well have been the cause all along. It's hard to come to terms with the fact that the medical professionals got it wrong, and that maybe I should have listened to my body. Instead, I didn't have time to keep digging or the confidence to tell the pros how to do their jobs. I had a life to live and ambitions to attend to, and the experts kept telling me the pain was just something I needed to live with.

Dr. Orbuch and I spoke for over an hour—not the usual fifteen minutes allotted by insurance providers for these appointments. We discussed my symptoms dating back to when I was a teenager. "Is this the pain you feel during sex?" she asked during my internal exam. I jumped in agony. "That's endo," she said.

In my twenty years of visiting various professionals, no one ever found the pain I feel with such precision. It was obvious that Dr. Orbuch knew what she was talking about.

We discussed surgery; the only way to actually diagnose endo-metriosis is a biopsy. I was afraid the same thing would happen as almost fifteen years before. "What if you don't find anything?" I asked. "I'll find something," she said, and she smiled confidently.

It's a bittersweet feeling to finally name what ails you after so long. On one hand, it's a relief because you can finally take ac-tion. On the other, endometriosis can feel overwhelming. There isn't enough useful information about it, nothing that encapsu-lates its all-encompassing nature or defines the all-involving path to recovery—except this book, which is mind-blowingly relatable, relieving, and helpful.

Endo doesn't just affect the pelvic region. The body's response to the inflammation it causes sensitizes the central nervous system, and if you don't know what's going on—as I didn't—this sensitiza-tion fucks with your head. If your head's not right, there's a good chance you're in distress. This is where endo crosses the line from a physical ailment to an emotional one too.

On the physical level, learning to live with the pain during most of my adult life compromised my pelvic floor. Without knowing it, I was compensating for the movement of organs over decades and developing postural habits to avoid painful intercourse. At the same time, I was also putting up with excruciating periods and bowel movements, chalking it up to the fact that I was a busy, stressed, ambitious person.

By the time I met Dr. Orbuch, I was at my wit's end. But being able to talk with her, to ask questions and receive answers, was the beginning of a new chapter. I never looked back.

First, she asked me to change my diet and start seeing a physi-cal therapist regularly. Let me be honest. I balked. I was a healthy woman who regularly exercised. What difference would a new diet and more money spent on physical therapy make? Let me save anyone from having the same doubts: WHAT SHE ADVISED HELPED! Sticking to an anti-inflammatory, low-potassium, low-acid, dairy-free diet hugely lessened my random pelvic burning and meant almost no pain during intercourse. I didn't do the physical therapy, because I didn't believe it would work. That came later. Again, please learn from my mistakes: Do it immediately!

On December 17, 2018, I underwent excision surgery. Four hours and five incisions later, I woke up to discover that fourteen pieces of endometriosis, ranging in diameter from two millimeters to two centimeters, had been pulled out of my abdomen. Endo had grown as far up as my diaphragm. It was so invasive that some implants had obliterated the cul-de-sac between my cervix and rectum, pushing my uterus all the way to the left side of my pelvis. My case is certainly not the worst I've heard of, but it explained a lot about the pain and discomfort—not to mention the emotional stress—I'd suffered from for the past twenty years.

Afterward, Dr. Orbuch insisted on physical therapy. Physical therapy is imperative after shoulder, knee, or any surgery. What's the difference? My body formed physical habits to fight the pain and it needed realignment. My organs, particularly my colon and uterus, had been pushed to places they did not belong. I needed help.

That was when I met Amy Stein. I walked into her office a week after surgery and burst into tears.

"I feel like everything is falling apart and this is never going to end," I cried as I fell into her arms. "I don't know why I'm here. I don't like physical therapy. I can just breathe and meditate through this, my boyfriend is being weird, my whole family is here for Christmas, the pain won't go away, and every time I think about something I have a surge of anxiety that rushes from my groin all the way up to my heart." I kept crying.

She hugged me, which I don't think is required for her job, but I am sure has become a staple of it. She worked on the parts of my body she could at that time, told me this was all normal, and explained the importance of a holistic approach to the recovery. I saw her every week, and she started doing deeper and deeper work. I began implementing her exercises, and slowly, the internal pain lessened. My work with Amy Stein was IMPERATIVE to my recovery. Physical therapy realigned my body after decades of damage.

Two and a half months out of surgery, I was remarkably better. For the first time in more than a decade, I had a pain-free bowel movement during my period. It's one of those little victories I can't scream about on the subway, but those of us reading this book will understand. It's a big deal to take a dump without feeling like a knife is stabbing you through the groin and you want to vomit all over your bathroom floor.

It wasn't until this recovery process that I realized how pervasive this condition truly is. It affected EVERYTHING in my life. I don't want to blame it for all my problems, but having a condition you don't know about for twenty years plays a huge part in making you feel out of alignment, not just physically, but also mentally, emotionally, and spiritually.

It's simple: To fight this all-encompassing condition, recovery has to be all-encompassing as well.

That's where this book comes in. It doesn't just outline a plan to beat endo; it's also a manual for helping women feel less alone.

I used to be scared of talking about my endometriosis. My greatest sadness, and probably the most costly to my sanity, was this self-inflicted shame. I didn't know how to talk about what I was feeling without having a name for it, and so I stopped talking about it altogether.

Endo might be an "invisible disease," but that should not mean that those of us who have it must also become invisible. It's important to talk about it, to destigmatize pelvic pain, and to look toward solutions. *Beating Endo* is a way to start that conversation, not just to educate those of us with endo about how to survive it, but also to educate our friends, partners, and families. The more people know, the less stigma there is, and the less stigma there is, the more of us will be able to beat endo.

SUSAN YEAGLEY

I watched my husband back out of our driveway as our little chestnut-haired boy waved from the back seat of the car. "I'm sorry you are hurting again, Mommy—I'm sorry you have to miss the baseball game," he said. "We'll call you when the Dodgers score."

And just like that . . . the car made its way down the cherry-blossomed street without me, once again.

I kept waving to my son and husband, while desperately clutching the bright red hot water bottle tucked into the waistband of my sweatpants. It was another month and another horrible, terrible, god-awful menstrual period.

I had become so reliant, so sickly dependent, on my almost a dozen heating pads and water bottles, I couldn't imagine going anywhere without them. They provided temporary relief from my painful cramps but couldn't soothe my confused head and broken heart. I was sick and tired of hurting. How many more games, practices, ski trips, teacher conferences, birthday parties, weddings, and date nights was I going to miss from this otherworldly pain? Was there no end to this torture?

At forty-seven years old, I was turning into the frog submerged in boiling water. The frog sits and sits as the heat is turned up

5 degrees every day until one day it realizes it's about to become the soup *du jour.*

Like the frog, I just kept rising up—raising the ceiling for dealing with my pain until I was absolutely boiling over.

My rock bottom came when I was driving my mom and son around Melrose Avenue in Los Angeles. We'd just finished a cake-decorating class and were reliving every delicious detail. As we laughed and joked about our fondant and icing trays, I suddenly felt a strong jolt in my right side. Holy God! This was debilitatingly painful. Like a fierce electric shock.

I had to pull over, stomach throbbing, because of an INSANE amount of pressure in my right abdomen. Yanking the car over to a side street, I hobbled out and collapsed in the grass of someone's front yard. It was a small, beige-brick 1970s house. I couldn't help but look in the window and see a nice family sitting down to a chicken lunch. I was wiggling in their front yard, ten feet away from where they were eating. They stared at me in horror—like I was a crazy person.

I grabbed my stomach. Something was bursting in my right side and I could not breathe. I was so embarrassed but in so much pain. My mom ran over to me, and through a panicky breath said, "Come on, honey. I'm driving you to the emergency room. Cedars is five minutes away."

When I called my ob-gyn to tell her that I was once again hospitalized for another erupted ovarian cyst, she said, "Susan, have you had enough? Are you done?"

I love you, Maria, for saying that.

Yes. Yes. Yes. I was done, but why was this happening? My ob-gyn had operated on me six years before when another ovarian cyst erupted. She cleaned up my ovary and removed more potential cyst tissue. I thought that was the end of my pain, but it wasn't.

The last ER visit was my final straw. I sat in my ob-gyn's office and had a complete meltdown. "What do we do? What's wrong with me? Why does this keep happening?" I begged for clarity, tears streaming down my face.

My ob-gyn did her best to answer my questions but recommended I talk with an endometriosis specialist. She referred me to Dr. Iris Orbuch. "Dr. Iris is the best person to see about endo," my doctor said. "This is her practice's entire focus."

Little did I know that this conversation would ultimately save my life.

Two weeks later I was sitting in Dr. Orbuch's Los Angeles office. For the first time in decades, I felt like I was going to be okay.

The first thing I learned from Dr. Orbuch was that endometriosis is incredibly difficult to diagnose. Many women begin to develop symptoms in their teenage years and spend their lifetimes in enormous pain, even risking infertility.

Traditional ob-gyns are trained to deliver babies and give Pap smears, so the mysterious workings of the beast that is endometriosis often fall through the cracks. Simply put, lots of doctors just don't know about it because it's so difficult to see.

But Dr. Iris Orbuch promised me that I would get my life back. And she was 100 percent right.

My surgery lasted close to four hours. Mine was a very severe case; endo had spread all over my ovaries, ureters, colon, and fallopian tubes.

Less than six months later, I was absolutely TRANSFORMED. My husband and child hardly recognize me now. I skip around the house, cook a mean lasagna, and have absolutely zero pain. I'm outside kicking soccer balls with my boy, at every one of his basketball games, and I'm the first one to stand up and do the wave at

Dodger Stadium. I am free. I am brand-new. I don't hurt anymore. I've donated my dozen heating pads and hot water bottles to the neighborhood yard-sale bin. Finally, I can live my life to the fullest.

Here are some life-altering facts that I learned from Dr. Iris:

> Women are told we should be tough and that periods are painful so we should just grin and bear it.
> Women are made to feel crazy and are deemed "too difficult" for complaining about period pain.
> A period is NOT supposed to knock you out of your life.
> 1 out of 10 women suffer from endometriosis. That's approximately 176 million women worldwide.

In the end, I was lucky. I've lived the California lifestyle for over thirty years, eating healthy—kale smoothies for breakfast— plus doing an hour of cardio a day, followed by meditation. I'm very aware of the mind-body connection and always sought out a holistic view of health and aging. It's why I was completely floored when I found out I had an advanced case of endometriosis. How, after all those gluten-free muffins and uphill sprints, could I still get this outrageously painful disease? What's the point of attending to my health if I'm just going to end up on a cold operating table?

The answer is that all that good nutrition, regular exercise, and daily meditation—all that healthy living—got me up off the operating table faster. My body was primed when I went into surgery— primed to take the hit and bounce back. Four evenings after my radical hysterectomy, I was sitting at my favorite restaurant in Malibu eating California rolls. I was truly astonished at how much better I felt. No more pain. My lifestyle made it possible.

I would tell someone suffering from endometriosis to make

changes NOW to support your mental and physical health. Go to physical therapy, visualize how you want to feel before and after surgery, meditate, eat colorful, life-affirming foods. Cast a large net to boost and support optimum health before and after surgery. Life is just too short to suffer from this crippling disease.

INTRODUCTION: BEATING ENDOMETRIOSIS

Remember the first time you heard the word *endometriosis*?

As with any new word—especially one so multisyllabic—you probably tucked it into your brain and forgot about it, until suddenly it seemed you were hearing it everywhere. Maybe a friend said it ran in her family. Or another friend said her physical therapist thought it might be the cause of her pelvic pain. Or someone said her urologist told her to ask her gynecologist about it. Somebody somewhere even said that her *nutritionist* mentioned it.

Then a few celebrities announced they had it, so for a couple of days, it was in the news and in the blogosphere—the latest social media meme. The sudden attention unleashed a volley of pronouncements: Endometriosis is all about bad cramps . . . Birth control pills cure it . . . Surgery cures it . . . Only a hysterectomy can cure it.

All untrue, by the way.

Yet despite all the mentions and myths, we'll bet you nevertheless will be shocked to learn that endo, as it is routinely called, is estimated to affect one-tenth of all the girls and women on earth.

Think about that. The next time you're walking along a crowded sidewalk, or are on a bus, or are part of the audience at a movie or concert or some other event, look around you. Pick out the first ten females you see and tell yourself that one of them is likely to suffer from endometriosis. Her suffering might range from mild discomfort to intense pain, from an occasional nuisance to chronic agony, from something she can put up with to something that stunts her life.

What *is* this disease whose symptoms attract the attention of urologists as well as gynecologists, acupuncturists, pain psychologists, and specialist surgeons, a disease that wears so many different hats and shows up in so many different forms? Since it is known traditionally, if at all, as a "female disease"—and therefore is not much discussed except in whispers—why is a nutritionist talking about it? What do muscle pain and physical therapy have to do with it? And if it does "run in the family" and is therefore genetically transmitted, doesn't that mean that one in ten of us are just destined to get endometriosis and can't do much about it once we do?

No. We can answer with certainty that while endometriosis can indeed be genetically transmitted, many other factors may influence its development, and whatever the cause, there is a great deal you can do about the disease. That is what we will tell you about in this book, in which we will arm you with the most powerful weapon you can wield to beat this disease and live the life you deserve—namely, the knowledge you'll gain in the pages that follow. Understanding the disease—knowing what you're up against—is crucial to beating the disease. It's the starting point.

We are a gynecologist and a physical therapist linked by a shared and passionate commitment to caring for the women and girls who suffer from endometriosis. We came to this shared commitment from different healthcare specialties, as you can see from the initials attached to our names, and we arrived at it from different beginnings and along different paths. Pretty much from the start of our careers as medical doctor and doctor of physical therapy, each of us found ourselves caring for female patients whose symptoms ranged from pelvic pain to abdominal bloating to painful periods to diarrhea or constipation to fatigue and depression to infertility. Not particularly unusual in either practice, yet in too many instances, the ailments did not seem to yield to the standard treatments our specialties prescribed. And while each of us focused intently on doing whatever we could with the expertise we possessed, we sensed there had to be more we should be doing if we were to achieve a comprehensive cure. Patients got better. Substantially better. Often vastly better. But not 100 percent better.

Until, drawing not only on our own expertise and experience but also on that of scores of other practitioners, we devised a multifaceted and integrated approach that beats the disease known as endometriosis, an approach that gets past precisely what was afflicting these patients. The approach does not *cure* endometriosis; there is not yet a known cure. But it does empower those who have the disease to keep it from taking over their lives so they can reclaim the quality of life they want and deserve.

We don't remember precisely when and how we first connected across the gap between our separate professional silos. It's a bit puzzling because the healthcare community in New York City, where both of us began our careers, is still a closely defined world in which practitioner names are exchanged swiftly and easily along lines of shared professional focus. We suspect that we might have been introduced to or encountered each other or at least have noted each other's name tags at a large and busy conference about pelvic pain, a key marker of endo. Or it's possible that a colleague known to us both suggested a patient referral to the other—a sort of secondhand and oblique connection.

But however vague its origins, what forged the connection could not have been more compelling. By the time we did finally find each other, the suffering that endometriosis caused in our patients was very much on both of our minds, and each of us had concluded that a new and more comprehensive way to confront this disease was needed.

Our individual journeys to this conclusion help explain how we were able to create the integrated, multimodal approach to beating endometriosis that is the focus of this book. It's a pair of stories worth telling.

THE GYNECOLOGIST

Iris is the daughter of a cardiologist father. Medicine as a calling was no abstraction when she was growing up; it was more or less the air she breathed. From watching her father at work, she learned what became a mantra for her own future practice: first listen, then examine. Hear what the patient is telling you, then probe the body.

Iris carried the mantra with her through college and medical school to her residency in obstetrics and gynecology at Lenox Hill Hospital in New York City. Along the way, she married a fellow gynecologist, and she had her first child, a daughter; a second daughter would follow three years later.

Meanwhile, her residency completed, Iris went on to a fellowship in Advanced Laparoscopic and Pelvic Surgery with Dr. Harry Reich and Dr. C. Y. Liu, pioneers in endometriosis excision surgery. It was an incredible opportunity to work in their technologically advanced operating room, but what made the fellowship really special was the tutelage of the two men who had made significant advancements in the minimally invasive procedure that is the only proper treatment for the disease—excision surgery that cuts out of the body the misplaced tissue that caused the endo and confirms the presence of the disease. Reich and Liu mentored the young woman who shared their passion for the surgery they had perfected. Like her father, they listened closely to their patients. Sitting beside one or the other of them day after day as they heard patients tell of their pain and indeed their fears became for Iris an unforgettable introduction to the very real suffering that endo inflicted.

In 2005, Iris began her own practice, often operating along with Dr. Liu in those early years. Like her mentors, she made excision surgery her signature procedure, and as both they and her father had taught her, she spent whatever time it took to listen to her patients. The more she heard about their debilitating pain, overreliance on opioids and other painkillers, bladder and bowel ailments that seemed never to go away, pain during sex, depression—and sometimes all of those things together—the more she committed herself to doing whatever it took to restore their quality of life.

The issue became even more pressing when Iris read about a study[1] that had tracked the long-term progress of women who had undergone excision surgery. The finding that particularly resonated was an almost passing remark in the discussion that even after "meticulous removal of all endometriosis," a number of patients continued to be "symptomatic." The removal of the endo tissue was not, as both patients and doctors had hoped, a complete cure. Instead, noted the study, "another cause of (a patient's) pain should be considered." To Iris, this statement struck a chord, prompting her to consider whether surgery alone was enough; perhaps more was needed if these patients were to regain the quality of their lives.

The study ignited Iris's intellectual curiosity even as it touched a deep emotional chord. The question seemed simple: *What was keeping these women from getting 100 percent better?* What was the final piece of the puzzle that would return them to the kind of robust vigor and well-being their age and their dreams required? The medical literature offered no answers, while research findings reported at medical conferences focused on technology and drugs—and seemed to Iris to miss the point. She reviewed patterns of symptoms that her patients told her kept recurring—rectal spasms, shooting pains down the legs, pain after sex that lasted hours and sometimes days and ultimately produced anxiety and depression—but was unable to uncover any explanation. The question haunted her. Despite all the firepower being aimed at endometriosis, why were women still suffering?

THE PHYSICAL THERAPIST

At a similar point in her career, Doctor of Physical Therapy Amy Stein was asking herself the same question, arrived at along a somewhat different trajectory. As a little girl growing up in a suburb along Philadelphia's Main Line, Amy thought she might like to become a veterinarian one day. College changed all that; by her own count, she went through five majors, eventually getting a degree in Spanish literature before going on to a master's in physical therapy. The doctorate took a little longer, thanks to her giving birth to two kids two years apart, and to her expanding medical practice—she opened her first private office in 2003, her second in 2018—and her growing prominence as a pioneering expert in addressing pelvic pain through biomechanics, manual therapy, and stretching and strengthening exercises.* Yet from the vantage of that expertise, she found herself puzzled by a particular group of patients whose pain did not improve further once they had reached a certain plateau.

---

* Amy is the author of *Heal Pelvic Pain*, published in 2008 by McGraw Hill; she has served since 2008 on the board of the International Pain Society and as its president in 2017.

Like Iris, who flouted much of standard medical practice by spending all the time needed to listen to her patients—well over the times "assigned" by insurance or hospital guidelines—Amy began her therapeutic approach by considering the whole body. To Amy, that meant hearing and, as physical therapists do, literally touching a patient's pain.

But also like Iris, Amy found herself perplexed by the group whose progress seemed to slow and then virtually come to a halt once they got past a particular point. She was disheartened too by the misdiagnoses and subsequent medical mismanagement she observed in so many of those patients. Most had been referred to her following considerable time in treatment by urologists, gynecologists, colorectal specialists, gastroenterologists, or orthopedists; some of them had undergone surgery—sometimes unnecessarily. Many had been diagnosed with irritable bowel syndrome or interstitial cystitis, as it was then called—painful bladder syndrome as it is better known today—or with urinary dysfunction or just with *pain*. Some had been told they had a mental health disorder. Many had been prescribed unnecessary medications that resulted in greater dysfunction, and far too many had been prescribed opioids that had brought minimal and temporarily relief at best—and which became problematic in other ways.

Certainly in most of the cases referred to Amy, whatever the cause, the biomechanics of the patient's pelvic area had been adversely affected. Amy's treatment of manual therapy, stretching, and strengthening—plus nutritional support and other self-care practices—did mitigate these patients' pain and bring them relief. But among the women in this particular group, the improvement they realized through physical therapy then leveled off; they simply stopped advancing. The very question that Iris was asking herself hung in the air for Amy as well: *Why weren't these women getting*

100 percent better? What was keeping them from advancing past the plateau? Patients would arrive at her office ranking their pain as 8 or 9 on a scale from 1 to 10—where 10 is the worst pain conceivable—and in time, the PT and behavioral changes brought it down to anywhere from 4 to 2. But it seemed that nothing she tried with these patients could eliminate the pain entirely. In her own eyes, Amy wasn't achieving the complete healing she wanted for them.

She was haunted by the memory of a 2005 meeting in Sydney, Australia, of the International Pelvic Pain Society (IPPS). Dr. Fred Howard, a prominent American gynecologist and a co-founder of IPPS, was giving a presentation to an audience of other gynecologists, urologists, physical therapists like Amy, nurse practitioners, and primary care physicians. The heart of his talk was a deck of slides showing different conditions in the pelvic area. "Raise your hand if you think what you're looking at is endometriosis," Dr. Howard instructed his audience. The pictures varied; some looked perfectly bland, some troubled. In all, some 15 to 25 percent of the audience raised their hands at some of the slides, yet *all* of the slides in fact pictured endometriosis at different stages of progression. It meant that 75 percent to 85 percent of the specialists and practitioners in attendance got it wrong or simply did not recognize what they were looking at. "Endo is being misdiagnosed," Howard concluded, and he added, "We have to make a change."

For the attendees at the conference, that presentation also made it clear that endo could only be reliably diagnosed via biopsy. The change Howard was calling for was for the practitioners in the audience to keep endo in mind when coming up against a puzzling condition in female patients—especially if the condition proved intractable and was related to their menstrual history.

Amy had for some time suspected that a number of these patients she was seeing might have endo, especially those patients who were frustrated by the recurrence of their pain, or by the fact that the physical therapy relieved certain symptoms while others persisted. She concentrated on making a concerted effort to raise the endo issue in reaching out to other practitioners. By now, in order to confirm the diagnosis of the condition, she was referring patients almost exclusively to the small handful of gynecologists she was aware of nationwide who seemed to understand endometriosis. At the same time, to address the pain in those patients who had plateaued in their treatment, she referred them on to the equally minuscule number of physiatrists she was aware of at the time—specialists in physical medicine and rehabilitation aimed at restoring function in the case of a disabling or chronic impairment. She kept making connections among these practitioners, introducing herself, via email or in accompanying a patient to a doctor's appointment, representing herself as a member of the Board of the International Pelvic Pain Society and asking to chat. She wanted to be sure there was a meeting of the minds before she referred patients onward.

TEAMING UP

We think that Iris received one of those emails and replied right back that she was convinced that physical therapy was a "huge missing link" in the whole pelvic pain/endometriosis picture. We think that is what brought Amy into Iris's office one day to talk about the work she was doing, the results she was seeing, and the limits she came up against. What we both know is that not too long into our conversation, light bulbs lit up in both our brains. Here was a kindred spirit—a practitioner on the same wavelength and asking the same question about far too many women who were not getting better and who very likely, in both our views, suffered from endometriosis.

From Amy's point of view, Iris was one of perhaps a handful of surgeons throughout the United States who did *not* think surgery was the immediate go-to solution for the pain and discomfort she witnessed in her endo patients. At last, here was a New York City medical expert—a prominent specialist in endo—who took a holistic approach. From Iris's point of view, Amy was a practitioner who actually brought pain relief to endo sufferers through PT techniques that managed the biomechanical and tissue dysfunctions, through basic nutrition, and through other forms of self-care—without drugs—and who understood that more was needed.

She gets it! Iris decided. *So does she!* thought Amy. In a kind of mutual relief, a professional partnership was born.

We had and have a lot in common in our personal and professional lives, but what binds us together absolutely is this shared passion for caring for women with endo. We have seen how the disease can sharply limit the scope of a woman's capabilities, curb her physical activities, restrict her opportunities for work and school and play, burden her spirit and emotional well-being, blunt the pleasure or satisfaction of daily life with family and friends, and diminish the most physically and mentally robust decades available to her.

Starting in about 2010, we began to mesh our specialties and to expand our portfolio of therapeutic resources. Our aim was first to understand the disease process in greater depth and detail, then to create an effective approach to dealing with it. We constantly talked to each other about what we were seeing and about what worked and what didn't work to bring relief. And we reached out to practitioners and researchers across the healthcare spectrum, exploring what they were doing that was pertinent. Their input became part and parcel of the integrated approach this book presents, and you will hear directly from a number of them in the pages that follow.

We also will take a closer look at the impact the disease of endometriosis can have on a woman's life. We'll note the treatments typically offered by a fragmented medical profession that often sees only through its separate specialties and fails to look at the whole patient, and we will show you why so many of those treatments fail to provide sustained relief.

What we'll arrive at instead is an integrated multimodal strategy that will equip you with the knowledge you need to begin to beat endo and reclaim your life. By "multimodal" we mean that our protocol comprises different actions; by "integrated" we mean the actions are purposefully linked in an individual "set" or "arrangement" that is right for you. It includes, when needed and at the right time in your treatment process, the excision surgery that is the sole known method for *removing* endometriosis from the body.

While we are both sympathetic to the contemporary reader's tendency to jump to the chapter that seems most personally relevant, we urge you to read the chapters of *Beating Endo* in order. Understanding the full implications of what this disease can do is the first essential for beating it, and that understanding unfolds almost as a narrative. At the same time, we put in your hands the tools to combat every theft of life endo represents, and we show you how, if you use the tools right, you can take back your life from the disease and live it to the fullest.

Our own bottom line is that no girl or woman need feel that she is defined by her endometriosis, nor should any girl or woman be robbed of her strength, her comfort, her joy in her own body, and sometimes her fertility by this disease. This book is our prescription for ensuring that.

BEATING ENDO

WHAT IS ENDO?

The Disease Process
of Endometriosis

The endometrium is the lining of the uterus. In an estimated 176 million women worldwide, cells *similar* to those in the lining of the uterus are found *outside* the uterus. In these women, the presence of those cells where they don't "belong" distorts the body's anatomy, ignites an inflammatory response, and increases the likelihood of autoimmune dysfunction and disease. The result can be a process of progressively accumulating symptoms—although it may not be; there are women with endometriosis who never know it and are never affected by the pain it can cause.

But if those cells outside the uterus *do* initiate such a process, the progressively accumulating symptoms can be wide-ranging. This is because the inflammatory response sets off cascading chain reactions of localized and downstream effects that impact the normal physiological functioning of the body. This is one of endo's distinctive traits. Its varied "spin-off" ailments affect so many of the body's systems: interstitial cystitis/painful bladder syndrome, pelvic floor dysfunction, irritable bowel syndrome, sensitization of the central nervous system, not to mention anxiety and depression from the physiological changes and the pain they bring— sometimes to the point of debilitation.

As a result, a woman with endo may see a range of specialists and receive a range of diagnoses, along with prescriptions for medications or procedures that bring no lasting relief. She is equally likely to undergo tests that return a finding of "normal" even though the woman lives every day in pain and discomfort, or to receive a puzzled non-diagnosis—remember the 75 percent to 85 percent of doctors at Amy's meeting in Sydney who didn't know endo when they saw it?

Maybe that's why medical schools typically have given it short shrift. If you can't see it and you can't measure it, it's hard to teach. And with a lot of medical insurance plans holding doctors to a standard fifteen minutes of one-on-one consultation per patient, maybe there's just not enough time for even the most compassionate of physicians to dig deep into understanding what might be going on inside a female patient's body. Let's face something else as well: The fact that it is exclusively a woman's disease may be part of the problem. It is perhaps why, in March 2017, the then-president of the American College of Obstetrics and Gynecology could report that "63 percent of general practitioners feel uncomfortable diagnosing and treating patients with endometriosis, and as many as half are unfamiliar with the three main symptoms of the disease."[2]

It is estimated that from seven to as many as twelve years pass between the onset of endo symptoms and its proper diagnosis, during which time the woman or girl with endo may undergo a range of treatments, some of them ineffective, some of them with side effects that outweigh their benefits. We both have seen women who had been prescribed multiple different narcotic pain medications, others who went through gynecological, gastrointestinal, even orthopedic surgeries that brought neither relief nor respite and that turned out to be needless traumas to the body.

So we are left with a great many women afflicted with endometriosis who simply do not know they have it, and with a great many others who assume it is just something they must put up with—part of the price of being female, nothing specific to put a name to. To a great extent, therefore, endometriosis remains something of an enigma—a disease afflicting millions that nevertheless resides in the shadows of medical science.

What is well known, however, especially by those who suffer from endo, is what it can do to the lives of the women afflicted with it. We know it too. We've seen it up close and personal. As caregivers, as women, as mothers of daughters, we can't help but feel directly affected by the suffering we witnessed.

If you have been diagnosed with endometriosis, or if you suspect you may have it, you should know that a positive diagnosis is possible only via analysis of excised tissue; it's what the medical profession calls "pathological confirmation." Short of that, there is as of yet no other test to confirm the presence of the disease—no image, no scan, no sampling of fluids. (In chapter 2, however, we will discuss some important signals every woman should pay attention to.)

For many women but not for all, the principal and defining symptom of endometriosis is pain. In some, the pain is minimal or intermittent or even inconsequential. There are also women who are discovered to have endo lesions—the visible evidence of the disease's damage that surgeons like Iris can see laparoscopically and excise—but who experience no symptoms and feel no pain at all. In too many women, however, the pain may be anywhere from difficult to utterly incapacitating.

Unlike so many other medical "conditions," the pain of the endo disease process does not progress in incremental steps from A to B to C to D, where A is uncomfortable, B is pain, C is worse pain, and D is disabling pain. An endo patient may experience all of those levels of pain, but it isn't always because the disease is getting worse. It may also be that the disease is affecting so many of her bodily systems concurrently.

Ask a woman with endo where and when her pain occurs, as we do, and she will locate it just about everywhere and at any time: around the lower abdomen . . . in the back . . . deep in the pelvis . . . on the right side . . . on the left side . . . worse during her period . . . worse during ovulation . . . worse all month long . . . worse before her period . . . worse after her period . . . in the rectum . . . down the legs . . . up the vagina . . . during sex . . . after sex . . . around the ribs . . . up into the diaphragm . . . during bladder and bowel functions . . . in the groin area . . . hard to pinpoint . . . everywhere . . . most of the time . . . all of the time. Some describe the pain as acute, catching them unawares, without warning. For others, it is a persistent presence. We've heard the pain described as knifelike, a feeling of heaviness, a hot poker, sharp and radiating. Like lying down on a bed of thistles. Can't find a comfortable position for sleeping or sitting. Can't lift my body out of bed. Can no longer imagine what it would be like to live without pain.

The variety of the definitions and descriptions, the potential ubiquity of the pain, and the lack of consistency between the intensity of the pain and the stage of the disease process or the "amount" of endo found are among the reasons this disease is so puzzling. For healthcare practitioners confronting women afflicted with endo, the puzzle turns this disease into a chameleon, one that changes its identity depending on which particular symptoms are presented and, given the highly fragmented nature of our super-specialized medical system, on which specialty is doing the looking. The same complaint can appear very different to a urologist, a gynecologist, an orthopedist, or a physical therapist, each of whom is likely to prescribe his or her own specialty's standard treatment. We call it "misdiagnosis roulette"—well-intentioned but confusing and ultimately both ineffectual and injurious. Talk to a urology specialist about bladder pain and she or he might plausibly diagnose interstitial cystitis/painful bladder syndrome or recurrent urinary tract infection and prescribe treatment accordingly—all too often, antibiotics. A gynecologist hearing a patient's symptom of painful sex might explore a range of causes—from a sexually transmitted disease to menopause, with a different set of treatments for every possible cause along the way. And for back pain, you're likely to be prescribed painkillers until the pain finally sends you to an orthopedist, who might recommend physical therapy for the back or even suggest surgery. Yet endo can encompass all of these separate conditions—and more—and you might undergo a series of interventions and take a range of prescriptions, month after month, year after year—to little avail.

That is typically what happens during those nearly twelve years between the onset of endo symptoms and its proper diagnosis. Twelve years is a long time to be in pain or discomfort, and it is a long time to be without an answer, without a plan of action, and without hope of a resolution. Why is this disease so difficult to diagnose? How does it happen in the first place? Why does it miss most women yet hit some women so very hard?

The truth is, when it comes to endo, the medical community has more questions than it has answers. But the one thing we are pretty certain of is that the lesions Iris finds when she operates on endo patients are the pathological consequences of that disease process that is set in motion when cells similar to those of the uterine lining grow outside the uterus. Since they're not supposed to be there, this prompts an inflammatory response, more or less the way any anomaly—an injury or an infection—prompts such a response as a defense mechanism. It's a little like what happens when you scratch your skin with a fingernail; whatever your pigment, the color of the skin at the spot you scratched turns a different shade. That's basic; it's Biology 101.

We also know what happens when cells form *in* the uterine lining because it happens on a cyclical basis, as all women are reminded once a month. Your ovary releases an egg and sends it toward the fallopian tubes. Hormones stimulate the uterus to thicken its lining in anticipation of the possibility of fertilization. But when sperm fail to fertilize the egg, the egg simply dissolves, and the uterine lining, along with some blood, flows out of the body—i.e., you get your period. All of this too is basic. It's Procreation 101—how the species keeps going—and most women's bodies are equipped to undergo this chance at fertilization every twenty-eight days or so, year after year from the time of our first period as a young girl until we age into menopause (except during pregnancy, of course).

The cells that are found *outside the uterus* are also stimulated each month by the same hormonal cycle. But these cells have nowhere to go; there is no exit point for them, so they get thicker and thicker month after month. In time, they distort the surrounding anatomy, and this can cause the organs in the area to stick to one another—the rectum to the uterus, for example. In women in whose bodies this process is taking place, the mechanism for clearing out the cells has altered in some way and fails to work. The cells accumulate, month by month, year by year.

Nor are endo implants limited to the vicinity of the reproductive organs. They can be anywhere—the lungs, the diaphragm, anywhere. Iris knew of a patient who suffered nosebleeds at every period; her endo implants literally were in her nose.

While we don't know exactly why these cells grow outside of the uterus, research suggests that there are both genetic and environmental factors that can put a woman at increased risk of developing the disease. If your mother, sibling, aunt, or grandmother—via either the maternal or the paternal line—has or had endometriosis, you have a sevenfold to tenfold greater chance of developing endo than the rest of the female population. That's the genetic factor in spades.

Other research, in the form of fetal autopsy studies, shows that an estimated 9 percent of female fetuses have endometriosis.[3] The suspicion of the scientists who performed this research is that either the fetuses inherited the endo cells from their mothers (the genetic factor) or that the fetuses were exposed *in utero* to a family of chemicals called dioxins (this is the environmental factor). Dioxins are highly toxic compounds found both in the food chain and in by-products of household and gardening or "lawn care" products, and they have long been identified as a cause of endometriosis. If a mother is exposed to dioxins while pregnant, her fetus is exposed to their damaging effects as well.

Meanwhile, the process continues. The consistently thickening endo cells take on a life of their own. They need blood to grow, so they keep on increasing their blood supply. They also go deeper as they grow, and as Iris explains it to patients, they act like Velcro, adhering to whatever is adjacent: the bowel, the bladder, the ovaries, the fallopian tubes. And since each monthly hormonal stimulation continues to fuel endo's growth and expansion, there's no stopping the process until a surgeon like Iris excises the endometriosis that is now thoroughly implanted in the body.

Given the *average* twelve-year period between onset of symptoms and diagnosis, consider the potential extent and severity of your endo by the time you receive that diagnosis. If your endo originated during fetal life, those implants have been growing inside you for a long, long time, during which your body kept on adjusting to their presence. Maybe when you began to menstruate, your cramps were so painful that you had to visit the school nurse's office and ask to lie down—the likely onset of symptoms. If that set you apart from most of the other girls in your class—and made the school nurse suspect you of being overly dramatic—you probably still didn't suspect anything wrong, especially if your mother told you she suffered similarly agonizing cramps and said it was just "something we have to put up with." So perhaps it wasn't until as a young woman you confronted pelvic pain, or pain during sex, or infertility, that you began to seek "serious" medical attention. By that time, the endo implants had been growing inside you maybe for a couple of decades, initiating symptoms that appeared to different specialists at different times as different conditions. Undoing the impact of the disease at this point would be no small undertaking.

And it isn't just the implants themselves that cause harm. It is their impact, multiplied as they grow and expand over time, on the central nervous system. As the thickening implants gain increased blood supply, their nerve density also bulks up. More nerves means more sensory messages being transmitted to the central nervous system. More messages being sent trigger more receptors to respond, further sensitizing the nervous system. Each response sends out its own message of stimulus, so there are now more nerves sending more sensory messages. This process essentially becomes a self-sustaining feedback loop in which the number of messages and responses continues to increase, and the scope of sensation continues to expand.

The medical term for this "loop" is called upregulation—a process of stimulus and response that just keeps amplifying.

In due course, nerves carrying these sensations of pain over-whelm the central nervous system, which eventually becomes so upregulated that it hits an overload alert. And since those overload messages have to go somewhere, they branch out via the spinal cord to other available pathways. What started as the irritation of a single organ in one part of your body now spreads to other organs, muscles, and nerves in any number of locations. In other words, what starts as a small trigger can result in maximum perceived pain. Physical therapists like Amy are very familiar with the impact of this cross-organ sensitization. They know all about the effects of what they call "viscero-somatic and somato-visceral cross-talk"—organ-to-body and body-to-organ "conversation"—when muscles react reflexively to some ailment or disease condition that starts in one area of the body and moves to others.

The result of this cross-talk and of all the physiological changes brought about by the inflammatory process is what we call the co-conditions of endo—all too often, a cascade of coexisting conditions: interstitial cystitis/painful bladder syndrome, muscular pain radiating outward and upward and downward from the pelvic area causing pelvic floor dysfunction, gastrointestinal ailments leading to a likely diagnosis of irritable bowel syndrome or small intestinal bacterial overgrowth (SIBO) or both, a revved-up central nervous system—until the whole body feels as if it is on fire.

While the expansiveness of endo can feel debilitating for patients and can be confounding for doctors, the reality is that the way this disease manifests itself makes perfect sense. After all, the body is an interconnected network. Our medical system is divided into separate areas of study and treatment, and so we speak of separate organ systems, but that is just the expedience of jargon; of course there are no walls separating the systems of the human body. In fact, researchers are gaining more and more insight into the various mechanisms that mediate all the many interconnections in the body. What happens in one part of our anatomy often has repercussions throughout the body.

Remember learning about fascia back in high school biology class—the weblike connective tissue under the skin that more or less structurally supports the muscles and internal organs? It's like plastic wrap—very supple, totally pliant, but a completely connected net. Pull at the wrapper here, and the effect can be realized somewhere else, far from where you pulled. To see what we mean, take a piece of plastic wrap and wrap it around a smallish object like an apple. Then gently pull on one corner of the wrapper and just twist. The whole piece gets pulled out of shape. That's what the fascia does: one little pull, and everything is affected. In the body, a disease response in one part of the anatomy can send ripples of impact across far-flung other parts of the anatomy.

One very practical and probably recognizable example of this chain reaction is what happens when you have constipation—a common issue for women with endo. In many such women, it is likely that an endo implant on or adjacent to the bowel has distorted the anatomy, or that the inflammation from the endo has altered intestinal function, or that the nerves growing from the implant are intensifying your distress.

Nevertheless, the body reacts reflexively, as you squeeze and tighten or strain and bear down in an attempt, which is ineffective, to empty the bowel. The muscles you're bearing down on are all part of the pelvic floor, which, as its name suggests, is like a deck of interconnected muscles, ligaments, tissue, and nerves that sit at the bottom of the pelvis and support the pelvic organs. Because those muscles are all connected, that unsuccessful pressure to empty the bowel can have the effect of making you feel the need to empty your bladder, but you can't, so you squeeze those muscles even tighter or you strain harder, aggravating the pelvic floor and furthering the dysfunction.

But your pelvic floor isn't the only part of your body that is affected. All of that tightening—the scrunching of the body into what is effectively the fetal position—can send shivers of muscle repercussion elsewhere. It is the viscero-somatic/somato-visceral crosstalk in action: The body reflexively scrunches into a ball against the pain in the gut, and this scrunching pulls on the abdominal and pelvic fascia and muscles, which in turn forces rounding of the back and tightening and potential shortening of the abdominal muscles and, as the fascia web gets twisted ever so slightly, can affect other muscles in the body.

These multiplying and intensifying co-conditions are a central fact of endo, spawned over time as the central nervous system upregulates hotter and hotter and sends out more pathways of sensitization around the interconnected web of the fascia. The great majority of these co-conditions constitute morbidities in their own right—ailments and disorders with their own names and, often, their own prescribed treatments. They include not just the pelvic floor and gastrointestinal and musculoskeletal conditions, but also the anxiety, depression, and sheer fatigue that can follow as a consequence of the relentless toll of these conditions.

In most endo patients, these co-conditions have developed over the course of several years, if not a decade or more. If these co-conditions accrue so as to upregulate the central nervous system, symptoms are obviously exacerbated. And that, in turn, can obscure the diagnosis for the physician treating the patient. It is one reason that the disease is so baffling to clinicians of every stripe. But these co-conditions also offer critical insight and may provide the key to beating endo.

ADENOMYOSIS: AN ADDED GLITCH

As if all this weren't enough, it is time to introduce what we might call a "close relative" of endometriosis—namely, adenomyosis. Where endo is defined as cells similar to those in the uterine lining forming outside the uterus, adenomyosis occurs when cells similar to those in the uterine lining form within the smooth *muscle* of the uterus, as the *myo* in the name indicates.

Like endo, adenomyosis is hard to diagnose, although it sometimes can be detected via an MRI scan. The problem, however, is that if the MRI does *not* detect the disease, that negative finding has a 50-50 chance of being wrong. In other words, not seeing adenomyosis in magnetic resonance imaging does *not* mean it isn't there. So the MRI is not an ideal diagnostic tool, but it's the best we have as of this writing.

Detected or not, most women who have adenomyosis also have endo, and the two conditions share many symptoms. It doesn't work vice versa; that is, it is *not* the case that most women with endo also have adenomyosis. The particularly harsh afflictions of adenomyosis include very heavy periods, onerous lower back pain, and what patients call a "heaviness" and "pressure" in the pelvis. What the sharing of symptoms means, however, is that both these inflammatory conditions respond to all the therapies and practices you'll be reading about in this book. The two conditions, endometriosis and adenomyosis, are thus yin and yang—you really can't talk about one without the other, except when discussing treatment approaches. So it is important, in a book about endo, for you to know about adenomyosis as well.

THE KEY TO BEATING ENDO

Nancy Petersen is a retired nurse and an abiding icon of the movement for endometriosis research and treatment. She herself was a victim of what she has called "the mania of persistent misdiagnosis," undergoing multiple surgeries that neither ended nor assuaged her pain until she more or less self-diagnosed her endo and set out to change the way the medical community approaches the disease. She is the founder of the Facebook group called Nancy's Nook, a go-to source of information and a safe space for discussion about endo for, as of this writing, some 61,000 endo sufferers.

Petersen has spoken about the anger and "sense of victimization patients can feel when the system fails them," and about the need, as she says, to "get past it." Once you do, she also reminds patients that there is no single magic bullet for endo. "Meds do not treat endo," Nancy stresses; "they treat symptoms only." Rather, each co-condition—each generator of your pain, discomfort, or dysfunction—must be addressed with its own treatment plan. For example, "you cannot remove endo," she writes,[4] "and expect pelvic floor dysfunction to fully resolve."

What Nancy says informs our own approach to beating endometriosis—in an integrated, multimodal way. As you go through this book, you will gain the knowledge and understanding that can help you target every single one of endo's co-conditions—any and all of the multiple generators of pain and discomfort that you may be experiencing.

Next, through physical therapy and changes in lifestyle behavior, you will treat each co-condition so as to cool the body.

This cooling process has the effect of separating out the symptoms deriving from endometriosis from those deriving from the co-conditions. At that point, you should have a discussion with your endo specialist about excision surgery. Meanwhile, you will have effected key behavioral changes that can keep you healthy against a chronic, systemic, and complex disease process.

CHRONIC, SYSTEMIC, COMPLEX

Ever since 1980, when the Endometriosis Association—the nonprofit she co-founded—first reached out to women with endo asking for their complete medical history and that of their families, Mary Lou Ballweg has known that endo is a disease process of the immune system. For more than three decades, the research registry she initiated collected data showing that the families of endo sufferers contain cousins and aunts and grandfathers and other relatives afflicted with allergies. These included such atopic ailments as asthma, a range of cancers, heart disease, and autoimmune diseases like lupus, rheumatoid arthritis, multiple sclerosis, and diabetes.

The research registry was enlightening in other ways. Early on, it disabused the medical community of the flawed belief that African-American women were somehow immune from endo. The medical establishment of the time had tended instead to offer a diagnosis of pelvic inflammatory disease, PID, to black women. PID is a complication often caused by a sexually transmitted disease; the unspoken but stunningly racist assumption was that the underlying cause of the trouble was sexual promiscuity. The registry also undermined another long-held assumption that endo was a disease rampant among thin, nervous perfectionists—the kind of high-powered "career women," as one magazine put it, who postponed having children or, heaven forbid, simply didn't want to become mothers.

But that's the point of research—to identify and, when needed, to jettison dismissive assumptions masquerading as knowledge. And the research-driven, evidence-based fact is that any woman can get endo—without regard to race, creed, color, professional pursuit, or socioeconomic status. Period. That said, Ballweg's research does suggest that it is more likely to occur in women whose families are prone to autoimmune diseases and/or allergies.

Endo is a chronic illness, and that makes it very much a disease of our time. Up until the latter part of the last century, chronic illness was not top-of-mind when people worried about their health or the health of their families. What our grandparents and certainly our great-grandparents were concerned about was infectious disease. Back in the mid-twentieth century, polio was the scourge that led parents to deny their kids access to the public pool in the summer, and mumps, measles, rubella—the infectious, contagious diseases that could run like wildfire through a classroom or school playground—were the diseases that kept our parents and grandparents up at night. Yet now we rarely hear the words; here in the United States, thanks to the development of vaccines and the implementation of public health policies, these infectious diseases have been virtually eradicated.

What afflicts us today is a whole new "class" of disease, the ailments we see dramatized in endless television commercials from the pharmaceutical industry hawking drugs for heart disease, high blood pressure, diabetes, asthma, digestive disorders, fibromyalgia, arthritis, bone loss, Alzheimer's, depression, and—starting in 2018—endometriosis.

Despite the fact that they manifest very differently, these ailments have a lot in common. For one thing, they never really go away. In many of them, the intensity fluctuates, so relief often seems temporary. And even the TV ads don't yet promise a cure (and warn of many, many side effects of taking the drugs to keep these diseases at bay).

What these diseases also have in common is that they are complex. They can exhibit numerous symptoms, and there seems to be no single cause you can identify for the existence or recurrence of your symptoms. They are the diseases we "just have to live with"—until there is a cure or they kill us. By 2011, the World Health Organization could report that what it calls NCDs, noncommunicable chronic diseases, cause more deaths worldwide than all other diseases combined.

Chronic illnesses also tend to be systemic. Most affect multiple organ systems within the body. Look at endo: Its symptoms can range across the reproductive system, digestive system, nervous system, muscular system, skeletal system, urological system, and endocrine system. It is accompanied by the numerous different co-morbidities of body and mind that we have just catalogued. It certainly looks like the endo disease process encompasses a lot of interaction within and among the various organ systems executing their various biological functions.

But how chronic diseases affect people is also highly individual. There are a lot of commonalities among women with endo, but each woman suffers it in her own way depending on her particular physical and biological profile—in effect, on her own genetic profile and environmental exposures.

So it seems clear that to deal with chronic diseases like endo, we need systems thinking and the kind of integrated, multimodal approach we'll be proposing in the following pages. To a great extent, however, the medical profession is still organized more or less around the infectious-diseases model. In that model, the aim was to find the organism causing the infection and develop a one-size-fits-all treatment—typically a drug—to zap it. This was a phenomenally successful approach, as the eradication of so many infectious diseases proves. But along the way, we got so specialized we stopped being able to see outside our specialty or to think in terms of systems or to look past the general to the highly individual.

That is beginning to change, as we in the health profession try hard to emerge from our isolated silos and look both at the way the whole body works and at the context—the environment—in which it operates. But if you or someone you care about suffers from endo now, you can't wait for that professional transformation to happen. That is why we will show you how to take charge of your particular endo by addressing its particular complexity—the symptoms *you* deal with, the co-conditions *you* experience, the tools *your* body provides you with not just to manage the disease, but to beat it.

One thing that means is that we will show you how to read your symptoms in terms of your own genetic makeup. This is essential, because the path to diminishing symptoms is through nutritional, lifestyle, environmental actions—all the tools of genetic expression—along with proper endo treatment. The science here is complex, but the takeaway is hopeful and empowering: If exposure to a particular environmental situation or lifestyle circumstance ignites a genetic response that is deleterious or painful to you, no, you cannot change the genes, but you sure as shooting can change your environment, your dinner menu, your behavior.

One of the very first clues to this came from the Endometriosis Association's research registry. Alongside the finding about the allergic propensities among the families of endo patients was the statistic that 57 percent of women *with endo* also suffer from allergies—to pollen, plants, foods, perfumes, cleaning products, a whole palette of sensitivities. Moreover, the reactions to pollen, the incidence of asthma, and the presence of eczema were considerably higher among endo sufferers than in the population as a whole. Most significant of all, the research showed that when the allergies were addressed, the women's endo symptoms also improved.

Does that tell us something? You bet it does. It suggests that women with endo are women with highly responsive immune systems. So it is perhaps not surprising that in 1992, Ballweg herself brought about the research that uncovered the breakthrough connection between dioxin exposure and endometriosis. She had learned by chance about an experiment testing whether exposure to dioxins affected fertility in lab monkeys. There seemed to be a connection, but Ballweg was knocked off her feet when she discovered that two of the monkeys had died of endometriosis, a disease that until then had not been spontaneously created in a laboratory setting. Ballweg sought and procured funding for researchers to probe the connection more deeply. The study she put in motion, exposing a set of lab monkeys to varied doses of dioxins, proved the point. The monkeys developed endometriosis, and those given the highest doses of dioxin were correspondingly most seriously affected. The conclusion was inescapable that "dioxin and other toxic chemicals can cause the development of endometriosis and other health problems to which those with endometriosis are susceptible, including certain cancers, autoimmune diseases, and heart disease."[5]*

This doesn't *just* mean that endo sufferers might want to refrain from using herbicides on their lawns next spring—dioxins being a

---

* Adding to the sweetness of having been the prime mover of this important discovery, the icing on the cake for Ballweg was that it happened at her *alma mater*, the University of Wisconsin, in its Primate Laboratory on the Madison campus.

by-product of herbicides. It's a reminder that the way we live, the things we ingest, the makeup and shampoo we use, the choices we make every day can shape the way we feel and the well-being we enjoy—or debase—every day. Beating the disease process of endo also has to happen every day, day after day.

Women with endo have a higher than normal likelihood of developing these autoimmune conditions:

Hashimoto's thyroiditis

Celiac disease

Sjogren's syndrome

Multiple sclerosis

Eczema

Rheumatoid arthritis

Systemic lupus erythematosus

Ballweg was a teenager when she first felt the symptoms of what she later learned was endometriosis. She would undergo a number of surgeries for her endo, including excision. But Ballweg is also, by her own definition, "a health nut," seriously committed to firm practices of nutrition, exercise, and the like—and she believes unreservedly that her own integrated and multimodal program made the difference. Once restored to full health, she formalized the content of that program by creating a protocol that she hoped would help protect her daughter from developing endo. In 2017, Mary Lou and her husband welcomed their first grandchild—a healthy baby girl, born of a healthy mother.

The power to beat endo really is in your hands. We'll tell you how.

Classic Endo Myths

Hysterectomy is a cure for endometriosis.
FALSE. Hysterectomy is neither a treatment nor a cure. By defi-nition, endo consists of cells similar to those in the lining of the uterus but found *outside* the uterus; removing the uterus ignores the cells outside. Only surgical excision removes endometriosis cells.

Medical menopause is a cure for endometriosis.
FALSE. Just because your medicines give you hot flashes doesn't mean your endometriosis is going away.

Teenagers are too young to have endometriosis.
FALSE. Teenage girls *can* have endo, and their endo can be at an advanced stage.

Pregnancy is a cure for endometriosis.
FALSE. Just no: Pregnancy does not cure endo.

Birth control is a cure for endometriosis.
FALSE. Birth control and other medical treatments treat symp-toms only. They do not cure endo; in fact, the endo keeps pro-gressing while you take birth control or other medicines.

If you have minimal endometriosis, you should have minimal symptoms.
FALSE. There is no correlation between the amount of endo-metriosis and the severity of your symptoms.

Endometriosis is found only in your pelvis.
FALSE. Endo may be found in many areas outside the pelvis. Lis-ten to your body.

Ablation surgery is equal to excision surgery.

FALSE. Not even close. We will explore this more in chapter 11.

All I need is an operation and all my endo symptoms will disappear.

All I need is to become a vegan and all my endo symptoms will disappear.

All I need is to take a few physical therapy sessions and all my endo symptoms will disappear.

FALSE. To beat endo, you need an integrated, multimodal approach—a set of actions.

THE GOAL

Regaining Quality of Life

We all pretty much know what a *disease* is; it's a disorder in any living thing that impairs the normal functioning of the area it affects and that may be manifested in various symptoms. But what do we mean when we talk about "a disease process"? It is probably enough to say that a *disease process* is a disease that keeps going. The impairing disorder with its various symptoms continues, and as it continues, it disrupts the normal functioning of other parts of the body too.

The pain generated by the disease also expands, upregulating an ever-wider range of the central nervous system and bringing pain to more areas of the body. A colleague of ours, urogynecologist Dr. Charles Butrick, the first of the other expert practitioners we promised you would be hearing from in the course of this book, puts it this way: "The longer the pain has been present, the greater the likelihood that new pain generators will develop." This describes the disease process of endometriosis to a T.

How do you beat a chronic and systemic disease process once it has been set in motion? By setting in motion another process that is equally chronic and equally systemic. That means, simply put, that you must be prepared to address the disease across a number of different organ systems; it also means you can't assume that having done so, you are also done with this disease. You won't cure your endo, but you will beat it. And that is how you will regain the life you want and deserve.

Our integrated, multimodal approach is such a process. But because endo can affect individual women in so many ways and at varying levels of intensity, the way you employ the approach will depend on your particular experience. For many patients, excision surgery to rid the body of the endo implants that have been causing pain and dysfunction is key. But surgery does not fully end the pain and dysfunction. Both have been part of your body for so long and have so upregulated your central nervous system that virtually your entire body and in a sense your entire life almost literally resonate with the disease. That is why it is so important to suss out each dimension—each co-condition—of your disease comprehensively and comprehensibly, preferably under the guidance of an endo specialist.

We are all too aware, however, that finding such a specialist can be a challenge. Our friend and colleague Heather Guidone of the Center for Endometriosis Care estimates that as of this writing, there are about one hundred endometriosis specialists skilled in excision surgery across the United States and fewer than one hundred elsewhere in the world. The reasons for these low population figures are fairly obvious: The excision surgery is technically challenging and requires advanced training—well beyond the basic surgeries most generalist ob-gyn physicians master during a four-year residency. The advanced training for endometriosis represents yet more time "in school."

Still, one of the authors of this book is an endo specialist who went through the advanced training, mastered the surgery, and writes from a deep well of experience and knowledge. So there *are* endo specialists to find, and probably the best place to find them is on Nancy's Nook Endometriosis Education, the Facebook group founded by the endo expert Nancy Petersen, whom we met in chapter 1.

Once you've found the right specialist, you will need to bring to the discussion all that you learn in this book about the unique multimodal approach we have created—which is not a standard that is typically taught—and then you and the specialist will need to examine in depth what the disease of endo may be doing to you: to your bladder, gut, sex life, and, pervasively, to your central nervous system. We'll help you with that examination in the chapters that follow. Then you will need to lay out precisely how to combat those symptoms so that you can reclaim your life. We'll help with that too; it's what our process is all about. Your endo may be fierce, but it is not beyond your power to tame and control.

Healthcare practitioners like us would call the process a protocol—a plan of actions aimed in great measure at downregulating your central nervous system. The logic of tackling one facet of your endo after another is that downregulating the system even a notch makes you feel significantly better. Feeling better gives you more energy to get stronger, and every advance in strength makes you better able to take on the next condition, then the next, and in time all the other conditions that may be upending your life. Equally important, any additional recommended medical interventions—excision surgery, for example—will work better on a less stressed, less inflamed, stronger, calmer you.

The bottom line on this process of downregulation and up-strengthening is that it will require a number of changes only you can make, for they are effectively changes in your current lifestyle. You'll almost certainly need to abandon ingrained habits and re-think routines that have become second nature. You'll have to learn and instill new habits and routines until *they* become second nature. It will take time. It will take effort. Again, it may require undergoing excision surgery—the one thing you really *can't* do on your own—and a process of post-op recovery. It certainly demands commitment. But it's the way to bring your endo-battered body back to a level of strength and vigor that lets you regain the quality of your life.

How does it work? Meet three women who did it. Different ages, different backgrounds, different experiences of endo, and at different stages of life when they came to our attention and under-took the actions we recommended. But all three committed them-selves to it, all three effected the changes needed, and all three have taken back their lives.

Here's how they did it:

ELENA

At her first appointment, Elena sat across from Iris and announced: "I've been told I have stage one endometriosis and I have under-gone ablation surgery," a procedure in which the endo lesions are cauterized—"burned off" rather than rooted out. Elena wanted to know why, after all that, she still suffered what she described as "debilitating pain."

Iris well knew of course that there is no correlation between the amount of endo in the body and the severity of the pain the endo sufferer experiences. She also knew that ablation surgery is ineffective in ridding the body of endo and may only temporarily—if that—relieve a patient's pain. Elena had a lot to say about her pain. "I can't function," she began. "I can't go to work." (Elena was an administrative assistant in a hot-shot investment firm.) "I can't have sex without pain." (She was in a long-term relationship with a decidedly supportive man.) "I need to ask my mother for assistance to carry out simple household chores.

"Help me," she said. "I want my life back."

Iris began, as she always does, with one-on-one questioning. She asked Elena about her history with endo from the time her pain began—she was a teenager—to the present, age thirty-eight. Patients tend to become downright eloquent when they talk about their pain—especially patients like Elena who have lived with the pain for decades. They are well acquainted with it, and they believe they know everything there is to know about it. But in listening to what a patient says about her pain, the careful clinician needs to pierce that familiarity and draw out of the patient precisely what a doctor needs to know. Iris listened carefully. Then she went deeper.

She asked about Elena's periods, which both were painful and produced an extremely heavy flow with clots. Elena told of having to leave a party because her menstrual flow soaked through and stained what she was wearing; her partner walked closely behind her as they snuck out as quickly and unobtrusively as possible. The pain, said Elena, was in no way limited to the time of menstruation but was felt at different times of the month. Iris recognized this as standard; the pain of endo can occur anytime.

Next Iris wanted to know about what Elena referred to as "stomach issues." She had experienced these "issues" since she was a teenager, and Iris elicited from her that she consistently strained when trying to move her bowels and found it painful to do so. She also felt a squeezing sensation around her rectum, and when asked about back pain, said that hers was the result of a childhood softball injury when she triumphantly stole home and stepped down so hard on the plate that she felt it from her ankle to her shoulder. To this day, Elena said, that injury made sitting difficult—especially during the long commute to work. Iris suspected that long-term constipation and straining her muscles in response to endometriosis were really what was at issue in Elena's pain, not stealing home base in high school.

Iris asked about her urological function, which Elena hadn't even mentioned, but in response to questions, she told Iris that she got up a couple of times a night to urinate, urinated twelve to fifteen times during the day, and still felt pressure on her bladder. When Iris pressed the point, Elena recalled that she had had five "urinary tract infections," as she dubbed them, the previous year, even though her urologist told her no bacteria were found in the test.

Moreover, Elena could not tolerate birth control pills, which one doctor had prescribed for her cramps, because they worsened her migraines and she couldn't bear the pills' side effects. Also, she had already undergone a full workup by a gastroenterologist, not to mention a colonoscopy, with results that, happily, were totally negative—nothing wrong with her.

There may have been "nothing wrong with her," but none of the medical treatments she had undergone, including her ablation surgery, had alleviated her pain—no surprise to Iris. Elena was exhausted, and she was becoming depressed.

It was all of this that had finally prompted Elena to seek out a specialist. Her boss, a senior vice president at the firm, had heard about Iris and suggested Elena call. She made an appointment for a "single consultation only," as she made clear; Elena was pretty sure she wouldn't be able to afford going out of network more than once.

But she had never had a consultation like this. She had never been asked the kinds of questions Iris asked—how often she urinated, did she ever get constipated, her sex life—and that was before Iris even began to examine her! So she was surprised and extremely interested when Iris told her that the interview alone suggested that Elena was dealing with a number of systemic conditions—urological, gastrointestinal, musculoskeletal—all of which were super-sensitizing and thereby upregulating her central nervous system.

That was just for openers. As Iris went through her physical exam, Elena felt herself being probed carefully from head to toe, a probe that, from Iris's point of view, confirmed her original assessment. Iris could feel the tightened muscles that told her Elena had abdominal and pelvic floor dysfunction. She noted the thickened ligaments behind the uterus, in the small space between the rectum and the back wall of the vagina and uterus known as the pouch of Douglas; thickened ligaments are a typical clue for endo. The pain that made Elena grunt when Iris pressed on Elena's uterus confirmed the suspicion that she probably had adenomyosis as well—endo-like cells in the muscle of the uterus. Iris was convinced that Elena suffered both that syndrome known variously as interstitial cystitis or painful bladder syndrome *and* tight pelvic muscles. It was also possible, she surmised, that in Elena's case, the endo implants were literally *on* the bladder.

Physical exam, questions asked and answered in detail, medical history: The aim was to translate a patient's catalogue of symptoms into an analysis of system dysfunctions. For Iris, it was a way of decoding heavy menstrual bleeding, back pain, constipation, trouble sitting down, and all Elena's other symptoms into a template of coexisting urological, gastrointestinal, and musculoskeletal conditions. And in its turn, it enabled the creation of a systems-based plan of treatment.

For Elena, learning that what was undermining her life was a panoply of conditions that began with endometriosis and that now coexisted with it was a revelation, but the realization that she needed to treat all of those conditions was a lot to absorb—especially after the false hope of ablation surgery. Yet in a very real sense, Elena was relieved to see this great, huge colossus of unreachable pain broken down into separate systems and into treatable conditions—with a plan for each.

Affording it was going to be tough. At age thirty-eight, Elena was still paying off student loans. She had been the first person in her family to go to college, but even taking six years to do it—so she could work between semesters—didn't pay for everything, and she had had to borrow tuition money. On the plus side, she was good at managing expenses, and she lived with a partner who valued her health as much as she did. What Iris was telling her made the disease that stalked her life at long last something she could get her head around, something she might potentially *control*. It was the first step to beating her endo, and it was clearly worth whatever financial hardships came with it.

Buttressing that notion of control, Iris recommended a few first steps of treatment, starting with pelvic floor physical therapy—a specialty of the physical therapy practice. She gave Elena a list of such specialists, and Elena, a New Yorker, made an appointment at Amy's practice. The cost would go well beyond what Elena's insurance plan would cover; Elena calculated quickly and decided that the new sofa she was eyeing for the apartment could easily be put off.

Next, Iris turned to Elena's interstitial cystitis/painful bladder syndrome, giving her a blueprint for an organic, low-acid, low-potassium, anti-inflammatory diet. She also referred Elena for an ultrasound to rule out the possibility of her having an ovarian cyst; the presence of such a cyst is the only imaging finding that ultrasound can reveal.

Equally important was the education Elena got about the difference between ablation surgery and excision surgery. Iris explained why excision was the proper treatment for endo, and why ablation had not worked for her. "Ablation is superficial; it burns off the top layer of an endo lesion—the surface only. Excision cuts out and removes your endo." But even though excision is the *right* procedure, it should be performed only when the body has been sufficiently cooled down from the upregulation the endo has set in motion. Think of endo as the first domino in the row, Iris suggested; when it falls, it sets all the other dominoes tumbling, one after another. What Elena had to understand, Iris told her, was that she needed to address all the "co-condition dominoes" before she could return to the endo domino that had toppled them into her life.

"You think your endo is the cause of everything," Iris told her, "but in fact it's endo *and* its coexisting conditions. As we identify all the conditions and find a treatment plan for each, you will begin to downregulate your central nervous system, and as you do, you will feel your pain and discomfort diminishing. So start with the diet and the PT to begin treating the interstitial cystitis and the tight pelvic floor muscles, and come back to me in six weeks. And bring the records of your operation and your past medical history so I can learn more. I want to make sure we cover all the bases before we schedule excision surgery." Bottom line: Excision is the right surgery, there is a right time for doing it—after you've separated out and begun to deal with all the coexisting conditions.

Elena understood at once that she would have to postpone more than just the new sofa in order to pay for the surgery when the time came. It would not be easy, but it would clearly be essential. In Elena's pyramid of necessary expenses, PT for right now and excision surgery for soon enough rose to the top, displacing repayment of student loans, the sofa, and the dream Caribbean vacation she and her partner had planned. Health first.

When Elena returned to see Iris six weeks later, she could report that she was urinating less frequently and was now "committed" to her new low-acid, low-potassium, anti-inflammatory eating regimen. She had even recognized that tomatoes, citrus, and coffee aggravated her symptoms; she knew this because she had cheated slightly, reintroducing those items, which had produced instant reactions. Now, needless to say, she was "off" tomatoes, oranges, and black coffee for good.

A less frequent need to urinate also meant that Elena was getting more sleep at night, so she was less tired, so she felt stronger, better, more confident about what she was doing for her health. And while the first couple of sessions of PT seemed to have introduced a new and different discomfort, Amy had explained it was because her muscles were just so tight that trying to lengthen and relax them would leave her sore. "Ever have a massage?" Amy asked. "The same way a massage that kneads the muscles deeply can leave you feeling sore, this initial flare-up of pain is a message that what you're doing is working." Elena could sense it too; she could literally feel that her muscles had a long way to go to relax, and after seven sessions of PT, she began to feel that happening. Moreover, her PT team at Amy's office worked with her on her bladder and bowel habits, helping her to recognize when she was squeezing involuntarily so she could begin to un-squeeze and relax the muscles instead. They also urged her to start using a Squatty Potty, perhaps the best known of the so-called toilet tools—a valid extra expense if ever there was one.

She was still bleeding heavily, and she was still in pain, but she could see a glimmer of hope through it all. As Iris told her, "You're thirty-eight and have been in pain since you were fifteen. You can't get rid of twenty-three years of pain in six weeks, but the fact that you're noticing a difference in *only* six weeks is promising: It means that your central nervous system is responding, and that this multimodal treatment plan is working. It won't happen overnight, but you can see that change is coming." Exactly so, and the glimmer seemed electric.

One part of the plan Elena had not yet had time to follow up on was to consult a specialist who could help her deal with her upregulated central nervous system. So Iris now referred her to a physiatrist who combined Eastern practices of mindfulness and meditation and Western advances in medical treatment to calm the central nervous system. Both approaches are needed, Iris argued. Learning how to meditate was powerful, but often not enough to cool the system on its own. Ditto for taking a pill: Pharmacology can be powerful but far less so when it acts single-handedly. Both together—meditation and the drug, Eastern and Western wisdom—are what cool the central nervous system and help restore the body to balance and efficiency.

The specialist alerted Elena that he would be starting her on a low dose of the medication he prescribed and would then increase the dosage incrementally. It meant she would not feel the drug's effects for at least a month, maybe longer, as she worked her way up to that "therapeutic" level of intake. Too much of this medication too soon, the specialist warned Elena, could cause unpleasant and serious side effects. He also advised her to download a mindfulness app and spend ten minutes in mindfulness-based stress reduction each morning. She would at least start her day in a downregulated frame of mind and body—"Almost as good as an island vacation," she told herself. But the specialist also recommended she start a serious meditation practice and/or begin seeing a talk therapist or pain psychologist.

Having experienced the benefits of her efforts so far, Elena embraced these ideas. She also felt she had gained a clearer picture of the multiple different causes of her pain. What she had thought was her "stage one endo" she now recognized as multiple coexisting conditions. She was beginning to understand in the most immediate terms how different actions raised the heat of her central nervous system. But she also wanted to know when she could have surgery.

"I could operate on you tomorrow," Iris replied, "but I would be a really bad doctor if I did that. I would be doing you a disservice. Let's cool your body down a bit more and wait about six to twelve weeks before we schedule your surgery. Continue the PT regularly, stay true to the diet, take the meds and do the mindfulness practices the physiatrist prescribed, and you will be well primed for surgery."

An administrative assistant working for a high-profile senior vice president at a high-profile investment firm doesn't get that much time off. Iris said Elena would need a week away from the office for surgery and rest at home (not to mention real healing, which can take as much as three months)—so Elena and her boss had to do some fancy stepping to get her the stretch of healthcare leave she needed for her excision surgery. It took another four months. The time was not wasted. Elena kept at the treatment plans for all of the coexisting conditions she and Iris had identified, and she saw dramatic progress in all of them except one: Her painful periods persisted—further indication that her endometriosis needed to be addressed by surgery. But she could sit comfortably now, only had her sleep interrupted "once a night at most" to urinate, and no longer strained as she once had to move her bowels.

She was also far less anxious, and each diminution of her pain, each easing of her body's tightness reinforced that equanimity and strengthened her commitment to the changes she was undertaking. By the time she finally had her surgery, the nutritional principles and the exercise regimen, the mindfulness and movement practices that had once been lessons to learn had become second nature—automatic behaviors intrinsic to her lifestyle.

In a way, Elena was lucky to feel improvements right from the get-go—as soon as she undertook those first changes in diet and began PT with Amy. The belief that the program worked, as sweeping and constant as were its requirements, was the impetus to keep going. The woman who had walked into Iris's office in utter despair had achieved a state of well-being that had previously seemed beyond reach.

TAYLOR

Taylor is twenty-eight, with a razor-sharp mind and a fit body, both of which she exercises regularly and intensively. A committed professional, clearly on the partner track in the law firm that snapped her up right out of law school, she works long hours and, given that her specialty is tax law, often deals with stressed-out clients. It suits her. She supplements—or perhaps counters—her work life with a highly active social life and frequent dating. She hopes to marry and have children one day.

But Taylor has persistent aches and pains. Once a month, she deals with fairly severe menstrual pain by loading up on Advil, which helps. But it isn't just menstrual cramps; she feels pain in her very bones. One is a frequent ache in her left hip. Another is an almost constant pain in her tailbone. In fact, she felt so uncomfortable sitting at a desk or at the conference table all day that she had a stand-up desk installed in her office; now her tailbone hurts only during meetings around the conference table. She finds that she must frequently bolt out of those meetings and head to the ladies' room to deal with an increasingly urgent need to move her bowels, and at the same time, oddly enough, she is beginning to realize that her "system" seems to alternate between constipation and diarrhea. Worst of all, however, is that she is finding sex painful. It started out as superficial pain, but the pain deepened and persisted; it has now reached the point where she finds the pain—both during and after sex—hard to bear.

She had been to see her gynecologist about much of this. His recommendation was that she have a glass of wine and maybe do some gentle yoga. Taylor already drinks wine and does yoga, although not the gentle kind, so she didn't find this advice terribly useful.

She decided to see an orthopedist about her hip pain and the pain she felt while seated. He ordered a diagnostic imaging test, and sure enough, it showed a labral tear in Taylor's left hip. What a relief it was actually to stare at the image of what was causing her pain! Despite the surgeon's warning that it would take six months to heal completely, she went ahead with the labral tear surgery and then began six months of hip PT geared specifically toward full recovery.

The operation was deemed a success by her orthopedic surgeon. That is, the labral tear was successfully repaired, and Taylor enjoyed slight relief from her hip pain. But the relief was minimal in comparison to all the other discomforts that remained with her—the menstrual cramps, her problems with her bowels, the tailbone pain that she felt sure would recede along with the hip pain but that did not. Above all, she was still having pain during sex. In fact, it was getting worse, and it was making her anxious and depressed.

Taylor tried another gynecologist. Sitting in his office, watching him take copious notes as she answered his questions, she noticed a book on the shelf behind him: *Heal Pelvic Pain*, it was called, by Amy Stein. She got her hands on a copy and began doing the exercises it offered.

She started to feel better, and Taylor expected that, along with the running and CrossFit that were her normal fitness routine, the pain would recede.

It did, and the bowel urgency also improved, but not enough. And the pain during sex persisted, which was extremely discouraging. Taylor wanted a cure; she also wanted a real diagnosis. She worked so hard at becoming fit and strong and healthy. Being a "healthy person" was a big part of her identity, and the inability to heal her symptoms was emotionally as well as physically painful. There had to be something wrong.

So Taylor made an appointment with the author of *Heal Pelvic Pain* and proceeded to Amy's midtown office. She narrated her story, answered Amy's many questions, and told her what the gynecologist had "prescribed." Amy was pretty convinced she was hearing the classic symptoms of probable endometriosis—and, in the gynecologist's "prescription" for a glass of wine and gentle yoga, an unfortunate bit of medical ignorance. After an extensive, head-to-toe external and internal examination with a focus on the abdomen, hip, pelvic floor, and tailbone, the pain points Taylor had complained about, Amy came to a far different conclusion and recommended a far different prescription.

She suggested a number of changes in Taylor's lifestyle. First thing, said Amy, would be to slow down the high-intensity running and CrossFit, both of which Amy was sure were aggravating the pain in Taylor's hip and tailbone. Second was a radical change in diet and eating habits: Amy suggested Taylor cut way down on the orange cosmo vodka martinis and focus instead on the bowl of nuts that accompanied them. "You need to go on an anti-inflammatory diet," she told Taylor, "but given your bowel issues, you also need to eat a lot of the right kind of fiber and to drink plenty of water along with that." She spelled out what she meant: "Everything organic! I suggest steamed vegetables and fruits, organic, wild-caught fish high in healthy fat—their omega fatty acids can lower inflammation—chicken and lean meat for protein, plus beans and the nuts." A change in diet, Amy assured her, could be the first step toward calming the bowel urgency and establishing regularity. For the menstrual pain, Amy was okay with Taylor continuing with the Advil for a while, but, suspecting that Taylor had endo, thought she might want to see an endo specialist. As for the pain during and after sex and for the hip and tailbone pain, Amy outlined a highly specific program of physical therapy—along with cutting back on the running and CrossFit. When Taylor objected to giving up her high-intensity favorites, Amy countered that Taylor needed "to let the hip and tailbone pain calm down. That's the first layer of the onion you have to peel off." She added, "Try the elliptical machine and a brisk walk—even a fast walk—instead."

It was a simple program: behavior modifications to downregulate Taylor's entire central nervous system, one upregulated condition at a time. Over the course of three months, she began to experience definite improvement, as she reported back to Amy. But she was having trouble giving up her exercise routine.

"Okay," said Amy, "but not giving up the CrossFit and running may actually be slowing the downregulation process. You're going into hyperdrive to burn fat and calories, and your body can't recover sufficiently. I really urge you again to switch to an elliptical machine in place of running. Just give up the high-intensity stuff until your system calms down, and in time, you will be able to slowly and carefully go back to it. Right now, instead, do some yoga, but not power yoga—the gentle form. And let me tailor a program of exercise for you that focuses on cardio, stretching, and some very specific hip and core strengthening."

This time, Taylor agreed to change her exercise routine, to continue with the changed behaviors she had already initiated, and to keep up the weekly PT sessions Amy had prescribed. Three months later, she felt almost entirely "cured." The two symptoms that still bothered her were the menstrual cramps and painful sex. Amy again emphasized that Taylor really needed to see an endo specialist and "get educated" about her disease process. "Not all ob-gyns are as knowledgeable as I would wish about what I suspect is happening to you, so let me refer you to a specialist." She referred Taylor to Iris for a full consultation and a thorough examination.

For a start, Iris did her usual thorough history and physical exam. In the latter, she discovered the same sort of thickened ligaments behind the cervix she had seen in Elena—plus a uterus tilted backward; Iris could palpate the area to reproduce Taylor's pain, and this confirmed her suspicion that Taylor most likely had endo. In fact, Iris estimated a 90 percent probability.

But since Taylor wasn't yet ready to undergo surgery, Iris first recommended birth control pills to subdue the monthly pain, cautioning Taylor that the pills would treat only her symptoms, not her endo. "The birth control pills won't keep your endo from progressing," Iris cautioned her, "but they'll relieve some of your symptoms." Second, and conceivably more important, Iris had an extensive talk with her about the disease she was pretty certain

Taylor had. She said she thought it likely that Taylor's endo was decreasing her ovarian reserve and could compromise fertility later on, and she suggested to her that she might want to consider freezing some of her eggs because, while fertility decreases in women without endo at about age thirty-five, women with endo need to face potential fertility issues at an earlier age—in Taylor's case, right now. Knowing this could be empowering for Taylor. "Come back and see me in three months," Iris said as she handed Taylor the prescription for the birth control pills.

It was a wake-up call, and it worked. Certainly, the lifestyle changes and physical therapy had downregulated Taylor's system, alleviated her hip and tailbone pain, and helped improve her bowel symptoms. Sex was less uncomfortable since she started doing PT, although deep penetration still hurt. The pill had also helped her menstrual cramps—she only needed a few Advil a day, not twelve. She had regained a good measure of quality of life by changing significant aspects of it. At that three-month follow-up, Taylor got a refill prescription for the birth control pills, a reminder that the endo inside her was still progressing, and a lot of knowledge about the need to seek out an excision specialist—wherever her career might take her.

For Taylor, along with the benefits of relief from symptoms was the reality of having to contemplate what the presence of endo could mean for her future. It was time to admit that she was up against a reality she could not dodge and a fact she might have to confront at any time. If her pain worsened, if her body responded in new ways to the disease process inside her, she had to be ready to respond with new strategies. Self-governance was important to Taylor; she felt good about all she had achieved in so effectively cooling her nervous system—and in general, in living a healthier life.

SARAH

Sarah, a transplanted Londoner, had suffered severe abdominal pain and disabling menstrual cramps ever since her first period as a young girl. She could not recall a single doctor ever asking her about her menstrual cycle. Finally, as a grown woman in her twenties still unable to get out of bed during her period, she sought medical help and was advised to undergo ablation surgery. That recommendation is the typical first response to presumed cases of endometriosis; it is as standard in the United Kingdom as it is in the United States and just about everywhere else.

Sarah underwent the procedure and felt some relief—at least for two cycles of her period—so she fully expected that the pain would continue to diminish. Instead it returned, worse than ever. Her surgeon examined her again and told her, "There is nothing else I can do."

Meanwhile, Sarah met, fell in love with, and married an American and moved with him to a midsize town in a midsize state in the American Midwest. Her pain, which was not confined to her menstrual cycle but persisted with no rhyme or reason, was becoming disabling again, so she made an appointment with a local gynecologist, who told her that while he could perform a second ablation surgery, he did not think it would work to alleviate her pain. Instead, noting her complaint of bladder pain, he referred Sarah to a urologist.

The urologist diagnosed chronic urinary tract infection and put Sarah on a course of antibiotics. Once again, the relief she felt was gratifying—for the three days that it lasted. Then the pain returned again, worse than ever. But Sarah finished the full course of antibiotics before she went back to see the urologist again.

His solution was to try another round of antibiotics, which this time brought virtually no relief at all. This prompted an intense round of questioning to compile more details in a search for answers. What the doctor learned from this was that in addition to bladder problems, Sarah suffered from severe constipation—and was unaware of it. She typically moved her bowels once a week, had always done so, and thought it normal. Sarah was now referred to a gastroenterologist.

The gastroenterologist prescribed a daily pill and a daily stool softener. As was now usual—expected, anyway—Sarah felt a bit of relief at first, but after four months, there was no substantive improvement in her condition.

A friend of her husband's suggested she see an endocrinologist, and an increasingly desperate Sarah made an appointment. The endocrinologist prescribed thyroid medication to raise Sarah's low thyroid levels and, having noted for years a correlation between endo and autoimmune conditions, confirmed the possibility that Sarah might have an autoimmune disease. And, since the word *endometriosis* was floating in the air, he also suggested that Sarah get in touch with a New York–based endo specialist—namely, Iris.

Certainly, Sarah had traveled a long way since her family doctor back home in England told her that her pain was something she would "just have to live with," so the prospect of a trip to New York seemed but another step in the journey and certainly worth trying. That was how she came to be in Iris's office, where she answered Iris's rash of questions, went through Iris's hands-on, extensive physical examination, and heard Iris proclaim that there was "a high likelihood" that Sarah had endometriosis. Iris also recognized that Sarah's pelvic floor muscles were extremely tight and sent her to Amy for physical therapy. Together, they prescribed a program for Sarah: It would start with understanding the disease process, changing to a low-acid, low-potassium, anti-inflammatory diet to address her interstitial cystitis/painful bladder, getting up and moving *and* beginning a specialized physical therapy program, moderating the disease's impacts one by one, undertaking a program of mindfulness through meditation, yoga, qigong, or tai chi—and downregulating the nervous system as preparation for excision surgery, when the time was right.

The prospect was daunting. But the alternative was unthinkable. If her suffering was needless, if she could beat the disease that was beating up her life by taking action, it had to be worth whatever effort, whatever programs, whatever life changes were called for. It was time to start.

After four months of physical therapy, a mindfulness program, downregulating her central nervous system, and cooling her body, Sarah underwent excision surgery. Post-surgery, she resumed her PT and continued her other new lifestyle practices—and regained her life.

There would be no point in asserting that for any or all of these women, what happened next was smooth sailing to a life without pain or discomfort. There was little about what each of them undertook that was smooth, and it certainly was not effortless. But as their bodies benefited from the new habits and practices, and as their minds gained the ability to differentiate among the sources of pain, the self-empowerment became palpable. They understood their own disease process, and they had a process for combating it.

Iris likes to explain it using the classic image of a young child accidentally putting her hand on a hot stove. You probably did that once, and if you did, you pulled your hand away immediately, almost automatically, as the nerves transmitted the message of pain via the spinal cord to your brain, which instructed you to get that hand off that horribly painful thing.

That is acute pain. It hurts, but after a while, it is gone. But while acute pain is entirely different from the chronic pain of endo, the image is still apt: Endo-driven condition by endo-driven condition, our program for beating the disease shows you how to lift hands off a hot stove. Endo is one hand on the stove. Pelvic floor dysfunction is a hand on the stove. Painful bladder is another. Anxiety and depression are two more hands on the stove. An overagitated, over-worked central nervous system, kindled by these conditions and burning hotter and hotter as the conditions persist, is yet another. To beat endo, you must lift *all* the hands off the stove.

As you do so, you begin to register *which* hand is being lifted; you recognize the nature of the pain and can trace its source. Such understanding is incredibly important to your well-being, because it puts you in control of your disease process. That is exactly how it worked for Elena, Taylor, and Sarah, and it is how it will work for you.

Can there be lapses? Of course. Both of us note a definite, collective lapse among our patients during the winter holidays—and an accompanying flare-up in those women's symptoms. Iris says it typically starts at Thanksgiving, the annual kickoff date for a month of not adhering to any diet plan and of drinking enough wine that patients stop caring that much that they are not adhering to their diet plans. Then they're too busy to go to their PT sessions regularly, says Amy, and their schedule leaves them little time for even setting out on a brisk walk. This is surrounded by all the legendary stress of the season, and all the expense and the pressure and the delights and occasional dysfunctions of being with family—right up until New Year's Day, when a lot of patients typically go on a health kick that can often be just as much of a shock to the system as Thanksgiving dinner was.

Remember: We don't promise you a cure. Not yet. What we do promise is a way to equip yourself in body and mind to overpower the disease that has been dominating your life. We promise to put you back in the driver's seat of your health and your future.

Ready?

ENDO AND THE BODY'S CORE

Why Physical Therapy Plays an Essential Role

What is technically known as the abdomino-pelvic cavity, the largest hollow space in the body, is bounded at the top by the diaphragm muscles, which separate it from the chest cavity, and at the bottom by the pelvic floor muscles. Inside the cavity are the body's urinary, digestive, and reproductive organs—instruments of life's most vital functions. Protecting and supporting those organs and their efficiency and effectiveness is an array of other muscles, nerves, tissues, fascia, and linking ligaments holding everything together.*

---

* To understand more about self-care techniques for the body's core, read Amy Stein's book *Heal Pelvic Pain*.

This is the body's core. It contains the muscles that hold us up-right and help us to move our arms and legs efficiently. Designed for endurance and posture, they're the hub of the body's motion *and* of its stability. The organs these muscles, ligaments, fascia, and bones guard are utterly crucial, determinative of the way we live: The abdomino-pelvic core is home to the agents of nourishment, to the control center of continence, and to the mechanism of sexual function.

And it is here that endometriosis begins, where its cells grow, and where—very often—a great many women and girls first feel its pain. To a considerable extent, that is a matter of geography. When the cells similar to the cells of the uterine lining form outside the lining, they often develop in a space located behind the vagina and cervix but in front of the rectum—pretty much at the deepest point of a woman's core. This space goes by a variety of names: the cul-de-sac or the pouch of Douglas or the rectovaginal septum; a doctor might use any one of those terms or all of them.

We'll call it the cul-de-sac, and just like a cul-de-sac at the end of a street in your neighborhood, it has no exit; the pouch of Douglas is a closed pouch. That means that as the cells of the endo implant growing there extend deeper into the pouch and adhere to adjacent organs, via the process we detailed in chapter 1, they eventually distort the anatomy of the cul-de-sac. This quite literally changes the anatomical structure of the core.

But that's not all. There are muscles underlying the cul-de-sac. The thickening cells pull on these underlying muscles and on the surrounding fascia and nerves, changing *their* anatomical structure as well. This pulling, along with the inflammatory response that endo ignites, is what causes your pain.

You react. It's natural. The body's response to pain and to antic-ipated pain is to protect, so your body reflexively tries to get away from the pain by tensing the muscles at or near the point of pain. If the pain is a menstrual cramp, you probably squash your body into the fetal position and tense the abdominal muscles, the inner thigh muscles, and the pelvic floor muscles. If you feel pain during sex, you squeeze the muscles around the vagina. Over time—for example, over the dozen or so years that typically pass between your first symptoms and a diagnosis of endo—the muscle tightening, squeezing, and clenching are going to leave those muscles and fascia tighter, less flexible, less effective in their job of keeping you moving, keeping you stable, and protecting the organs within your core. Your muscles will essentially be locked into a short, tight, and painful state.

And since the muscles of the pelvic floor are attached to the skeleton, it too feels the impact. Pull on your pelvic floor muscles and they in turn pull on your tailbone, your pubic bone, your lower backbone, and your hip bone. This can literally rearrange your skeletal alignment, which in turn can lead to backache, butt pain, and pain down the leg. If that happens, anyone watching you from across the room might notice that you are walking funny; you look imbalanced, and you are—your skeletal structure has gone off-kilter—from the pelvic floor to the back muscles all the way up to the neck and down to the toes.

Things start going haywire. From the pelvic floor at the bottom to the diaphragm at the top, everything that is supposed to work together becomes sluggish and inefficient. All the muscles, fascia, and ligaments that compose the outer wall of the core and all the organs and tissue within start functioning aberrantly. The body's natural state is to stay upright—vertical against gravity. If a muscle is pulling your body over to the right, something else will naturally try to pull the body back to the left to maintain that vertical alignment. As this muscular tug-of-war continues, some muscles work overtime, leading to pain, while others tighten and weaken. Connective tissue, which connects muscle to muscle and muscle to ligament, becomes restricted—its motion limited or impeded—so blood flow slows down. This means the blood doesn't reach as far as it must to nourish the cells and remove the waste—the very functions blood flow is supposed to execute. Muscles and nerves, bloodthirsty vampires, are shortchanged by this inability to slake their thirst; it's the condition we feel as pins and needles or when our leg is "asleep."

Shortchanging the muscles and nerves wears down the joints too; they don't slide and glide as smoothly as they should. And the vital urinary, digestive, and reproductive organs within the core, also supported by connective tissue, muscles, and ligaments, feel the distress and may become stuck or tethered in place. If they're no longer moving *with* your body as they should, they are not functioning at their best. The body becomes fatigued and sluggish from the widespread inflammation and the accompanying muscle pain. And the resulting impact on your ability to function at *your* best is unpleasant at best, painful at worst.

The unpleasantness or pain might start as a sharp or dull ache—or both together—somewhere, most likely in the abdominal wall or in the pelvic floor, right at the base of the core. And since the pelvic floor and its fascial connections surround the urethra, bladder, uterus, vaginal opening, vaginal canal, anus, and rectum, they all begin to hurt as well, as the message of pain shivers along the various neural pathways. After a while, it feels like everything hurts.

This is the vicious cycle endo can precipitate: pain, response, distortion, dysfunction extending throughout the body's core and becoming continually amplified in intensity—an ongoing loop of reciprocal intensification. To the woman whose body is thus affected, the pain can be sheer misery causing utter despair.

Pain in the Core, in Patients' Words:

"It's like a squeezing around my rectum…"

"I have difficulty sitting, especially on the long commute to work…"

"Shooting pains into my groin and up my vagina…"

"A sensation of pressure—like being pinched—right in my pelvis…"

"Pain and cramping in my lower belly, worse during my period…"

"Sharp pain or dull ache during sex—or even when I use a tampon…"

"My back and tailbone hurt all the time—and sometimes the pain goes down my leg…"

"It hurts from my abdomen on up—and sometimes I feel I can't breathe…"

"It hurts to put in a tampon; I haven't used one for years…"

"Shooting pains up my butt…"

"Urinating feels like sharp knives, and I can't empty fully…"

At a first appointment, many patients warn us, even before they sit down, that they probably will need to walk around during the consultation because it is so painful to sit; they apologize that they are "more comfortable" standing.

Both of us have literally touched this pain as we examined patients. From front to back—circling around the bladder, uterus, colon, vagina, and rectum from pubic bone to coccyx—and from the bottom of the pelvis right up to the diaphragm or the neck, where tightened muscles can affect breathing, a patient's pain and discomfort can manifest as hard resistance to even the lightest human touch. Or, with gentle pressure or directed movement, we can actually reproduce the pain and thus begin to identify its location and the organs affected.

The bottom line about endo pain is this: The tightened muscles and fascia must be loosened and your skeletal structure properly re-aligned right from the start of any treatment plan, at the same time that you even begin to consider medical interventions. Physical therapy is absolutely essential to beating endo. In fact, beating the disease will require a highly specialized branch of physical therapy, focused specifically on advanced pelvic floor treatment. Why the pelvic floor? To answer that, it will help to know something about the muscles of the abdomino-pelvic cavity.

For one thing, the muscles in this part of the body are mostly voluntary. That means that they're controlled by the conscious mind, not by the autonomic nervous system. In other words, we're in charge of them and have the power to undo impairment that has affected them. Second, as noted, they are skeletal muscles. This means that when we contract them, the energy of the action affects the skeletal frame as well, so reeducating the pelvic floor muscles is also a way to help realign the skeletal frame.

We also know that the muscles connected to the organs of the pel-vic floor—whether the connection is via fascia, muscle, or ligament—are mostly but not entirely composed of slow-twitch fibers, the kind that support your organs, prime your core muscles for posture and endurance, and stabilize your pelvis. The rest of the muscles in your abdomino-pelvic cavity are made up of fast-twitch fibers, which en-able short bursts of power—essential for controlling the opening and closing of the bladder (when you sneeze, fast-twitch fibers keep you continent) and the bowel, as well as for empowering sexual function.

So, these are mostly voluntary, mostly slow-twitch, skeletal muscles—all acting in their distinctive ways to affect some essential organs and to support an essential section of our skeletal structure.

How does endo lead to the tightening of these muscles? Suppose your endo has affected your gastrointestinal tract; in fact, constipation is extremely common in women with endo. As you strain to move your bowels, you tense and thereby overwork the muscles of the pelvic floor. Conversely, many women with endo have diarrhea and repeatedly squeeze their pelvic floor to prevent leakage of stool. Many have painful sex, which causes them to squeeze the muscles around the vagina during sex or even in anticipation of sex. The feeling that they have to urinate when the bladder is not actually filled causes many women to strain the muscles around the bladder in an attempt to push urine out. Over time, the muscles of the abdomino-pelvic core get so overworked that they are weakened, while the pain can seem constant.

Finding the right way to ease and relax these muscles, the very character of which has been "bent out of shape" in response to the endo growing inside a body, can constitute a complex set of challenges, and it is that complexity that spawned advanced PT practice focused on pelvic health. The training for it is advanced too, taught as part of post-graduate instruction and covering both a technical understanding of the challenges and supervised practicum in the skills needed to deal with them. Therapists thus trained can bring to bear a range of techniques and modalities—from finding and releasing both internal and external pain at the source, to actual mobilization of the organs, to neuromuscular reeducation and biofeedback techniques—that will, over time, bring relief and begin to undo the pain set in motion by endometriosis. These therapists are also skilled in educating patients in their condition and in empowering them to self-manage their pain and its treatment.

The goal of all these techniques and modalities is to ease the tension in the affected muscles, fascia, nerves, and bones. This easing of tension also helps cool the fiery breath of the nervous system, which in turn helps the organs of the body regain optimal function and start working efficiently again.

You may not need the entire inventory of PT treatments and techniques we describe in this chapter, but it will be helpful for you to know what they are and what they are intended to achieve. Virtually every aspect of endo that we discuss—and therefore virtually every chapter of this book—requires a PT response of some sort. So the treatments we describe here are the treatments you should expect to be prescribed to deal with the conditions of your own endo—and if these treatments are not recommended, you might want to ask why and/or look for another physical therapist.

Whatever techniques are brought to bear in your own case, however, be aware that there are no shortcuts here—either of time or expertise. As Iris says, if you're in pain and you go to a physical therapist who tells you to do Kegels or to squinch up your musculature in any similar way, you're in the wrong place.* You're probably also in the wrong place if you go to a physical therapy "mill" where your assigned therapist, no matter how well-trained and well-meaning, is required to serve several patients at a time—in one such mill, a younger Amy once had six patients in one hour—which means that he or she has to leave you with a heating pad or assign you exercises to do on your own for thirty to forty out of the forty-five minutes of your session. We both caution against that. The PT treatments you'll need if you're going to undo the muscular tightening that endo has caused require therapists with the proper advanced and highly specialized training in pelvic health and manual therapy. Such treatments also demand the right arsenal of capabilities those therapists can draw on, an environment focused on comprehensive

---

* Unless the tightening is a very quick part of a contract-release technique, as you'll see below.

treatment and recovery, and the dedicated time and attention—one-on-one and hands-on—per session to ensure that you are doing your part correctly, that the treatments are making a difference, and that you are progressing from one session to the next.

How to Find the Right Physical Therapist for Your Needs

Here are some key questions to ask a potential physical therapist—along with the answers you need to receive:

Q. How much one-on-one time do you spend per patient?
A. A minimum of forty-five minutes.

Q. How much of your individual time is spent treating pelvic pain and pelvic floor disorders?
A. At least half.

Q. What type of training in pelvic floor disorders have you undergone?
A. Three or more postgraduate courses—at a minimum.

Q. Do you use manual vaginal and/or rectal therapy? Do you prescribe a home program? What else?
A. A range of techniques is desirable, especially a home program, but manual therapy, both internal and external, vaginal and rectal, is an essential minimum.

And here's a final caveat: If, early on in your PT treatment, your therapist uses the words *Kegels* or *strengthening*, run! At this point, these are the last things you want to do to your body. In other words, understand what you're going to need from PT so you can assess whether what you are getting is appropriate and worthwhile.

WHERE, WHEN, AND HOW DOES IT HURT?

It all starts with an in-depth conversation and examination in which the therapist will do her or his own detective work to determine, simply put, what hurts and why. When do you experience the pain? During your period? All month long? With no rhyme or reason? Is the pain worse before and during your period and is your period typically heavy? How long have you felt the pain? Does it wake you up at night? Does stress make it worse? Describe a twenty-four-hour "schedule" of pain. What are the accompanying dysfunctions—for example, of bladder, bowel, and, if sexually active, sexual activity? Do you experience bladder or bowel frequency, urgency, retention, incomplete emptying, bloating, pain, or pressure? How bad is the pain you feel in your back, hip, or legs—annoying or incapacitating? What makes it better? What makes it worse?

Layer by layer, the therapist peels down to get to the source of the pain and to determine which areas should be the focus of treatment. As specialists, physical therapists like Amy and her team know what to listen for in technical terms when women talk about their pain. They know how to go *behind* the complaints about difficulties concentrating at work, about the inability to maintain a romantic relationship, about conditions that only worsen, to identify the disease process that may be underlying these problems.

To the profile they extract from these questions and the accompanying physical exam, therapists must add the specialized knowledge of what endometriosis contributes to this pain—a knowledge that must be obtained through individual research, articles, conferences, and other special programs. Unfortunately, even many skilled pelvic floor therapists are unaware of the impact endo can have on an individual's entire system. A number of Amy's colleagues, for example, skilled physical therapists all of them, expressed real interest in the fact that Amy and Iris were writing this book. "Endometriosis!" one said. "Great! I don't know how to treat it!"

Essentially, the right PT treatments and techniques for endo patients break down into four categories:

1. Manual physical therapy techniques to ease muscle tension, mobilize and release tissue and scar restrictions, improve the body's alignment and joint mobility, and enhance blood flow
2. Neuromuscular reeducation to lengthen and balance muscles and joints and to retrain bladder, bowel, and sexual functions
3. Therapeutic exercise for overall health and stamina and to maintain the benefits achieved in manual physical therapy and neuromuscular reeducation
4. Modalities aimed at pain relief or muscle retraining

MANUAL PHYSICAL THERAPY

Manual therapy is the therapist's hands-on kneading, stretching, mobilization, manipulation, massage—or all of the above—applied to joints, fascia, nerves, or muscles. The fundamental aim is twofold: to relieve pain, wherever it may occur in the body, and to improve the mechanics of the body by extending range of motion and enhancing mobility and stability. "Muscles are the pawns of the body," explains Corey S. Hazama, doctor of physical therapy and one of an elite group of certified functional manual therapists trained in specialized hands-on mobilization techniques.[6] "Muscles do the dirty work to protect the more valuable structures. The body will always sacrifice a muscle before putting a nerve, blood vessel, or organ in harm's way." That is, in essence, the body's natural protection hierarchy. When abdominal and pelvic muscles tense, for example, it's because they're protecting valuable pelvic organs and nerves. Those tensed muscles, however, give rise to the pain/response/spasm cycle that spirals continually upward, igniting more pain, more response, more spasm.

Manual physical therapy helps to release tension in the muscles, which in turn helps to dial down the pain/response/spasm cycle as the muscles feel less "threatened." By touching the muscles and connective tissue of the body in a precise way to quiet the tension, the therapy also opens a pathway of communication with the brain signaling that the muscle is no longer threatened and has been returned to full function; it's okay to move (more about this in chapter 7). This in turn allows the body to relax, realign its structure, and cool inflammation.

The overarching goal of this manual therapy is to start a new feedback loop—this time, of healing. In this new loop, the pain relief that comes as a result of the therapist's releasing and lengthening the muscles begins to downregulate the central nervous system, lowering the heat of the pain. Diminished pain lets the muscles function better, which means they lengthen further, contract more strongly, and relax when they should, and all of this can help downregulate the central nervous system even more. Pain relief and downregulation thus work in tandem, and just as pain once bred pain, pain relief now spurs wider, deeper pain relief and increased function. You've effectively switched the direction of that loop of reciprocal intensification—flipped it to go the other way. So now, the more times the loop circles around, the more effective the muscles become, the cooler the central nervous system, the deeper the release of tension, the more efficient the body's functioning, and the better you feel.

One way to enhance the effects of manual therapy is through the practice of deep, controlled breathing. Taking deep breaths that fill the lungs with air expands the abdomen and ribs and literally causes the diaphragm to descend. This motion massages the organs in the abdomino-pelvic cavity, encouraging them to glide up and down, which is how they're supposed to function. In addition, deep breathing reduces anxiety, relieves your pain, and increases blood flow, all of which optimize the healing process. Deep breathing is also a key stimulator of the vagal nerve, which, as we will discuss in greater detail in chapter 10, can be decisive in dealing with the pain of endometriosis. Teaching such breathing is an essential adjunct to the therapist's skills, and practicing it ought to be part of every therapy session—as well as of daily life.

THE TECHNIQUES OF MANUAL PT

There are seven specialized techniques a manual therapist is likely to apply to release the muscles of the abdomen and pelvic floor as well as the surrounding muscles. A good manual therapist can read the cues of the connective tissue of your body to determine the right techniques for you. There is not a one-size-fits-all solution; every individual demonstrates her own level of sensitivity, and the therapist must adjust techniques accordingly. It means that a firm touch, as you might be used to in massage, may not be the right technique for your body and could actually cause you more pain.

Myofascial Release

You already know that the fascia is that three-dimensional web that holds all the structures of the body within it; the prefix *myo-* simply stands for "muscle." A logical starting point for a session, myofascial release is a technique in which the therapist palpates the body to evaluate and identify—and then to treat—areas of tension or tight restriction. The idea is to extend the fascia's web, widening its area so that the tensed muscles it holds in its net can relax. The therapist uses his or her hands and sometimes a massage tool to find the restrictions in the fascia, then applies any of a number of techniques to release the restrictions, thus improving the elasticity of the fascia, following the motion of the tissue to release yet more barriers.

A common technique, *strain-counterstrain,** used with myofascial release, is aimed at reeducating connective tissue that has become restricted; it's particularly useful in "curing" muscle spasm. The technique is based on the principle of passive positional release, and it is infinitely gentle: The therapist identifies the restricted muscle in spasm, then shortens the tissue, easing the two ends together. This lets the tension escape and helps to calm the reflexes that cause the spasm. It is effectively a resting position, and that is the neuromuscular message the muscle now sends to the nervous system. The relief is typically immediate, and by holding the patient's body away from the painful direction of motion, pain-free function is in time restored.

Myofascial Trigger Point Release[7]

This is a targeted technique aimed at that knot of pain in a muscle we've all felt at one time or another. This knot of pain may be a result of a disease like endo—some patients in fact tell us it feels like the pain is in the ovary or uterus—or it may derive from more innocuous sources (like the pain in your neck from sitting in front of a computer all day, or the knot in your shoulder from

---

* Developed in 1955 by Lawrence Jones, an osteopathic physician.

carrying a heavy bag). Whatever the cause, that "knot" is a highly irritated spot in a palpably taut band of muscle or fascia that increases restrictions and diminishes mobility. What it feels like is the unreachable source of all our agony. An experienced physical therapist, however, usually *can* reach it, and while the pressure he or she at first applies can induce pain or tenderness, gentle kneading or sustained pressure in due course frees the restriction and alleviates the pain.

Trigger points, as the name implies, cause pain elsewhere in the body. It is why neck pain can travel to the jaw or cause a headache. And it is why trigger points that produce pelvic pain may radiate to the lower abdomen and make us feel the urge to urinate, or spread into the back to produce bowel pressure, or ignite a range of other impacts. The pain that the trigger point produces can be sharp or dull, local or radiating, deep or superficial. Yet once the trigger point itself has been released, any restrictions in surrounding muscles begin to relax as well. So it is not surprising that research attributes to myofascial trigger point release an extremely high rate of improvement in patient symptoms overall—83 percent[8]—especially, as we will see in chapter 4, in reducing bladder inflammation and pain; it can reduce pelvic pain as well.

Connective Tissue Manipulation

The therapist literally rolls the surface of the body, manipulating three layers of tissue—fascia, subcutaneous fat, and muscle—by moving one layer over the other, freeing one from the other, so to say, to release tension. It can feel like being pinched or like a fingernail tracking a pathway across your body's surface or even like something digging in under the surface. The tenser the tissue has become, the tighter the layers are connected, and that slows the blood flow to the affected region. When tissue is no longer pliable and blood flow becomes sluggish, toxins gather and get congested there, and that's when you feel symptoms of pain, numbness, pins and needles in the abdomen, the pelvic floor, the back, even down the legs. The loosening of tissue and the release of tension rush blood to all these areas and sweep out the toxins, leaving the patient with a definite sensation that something has happened—often manifested as an initial feeling of soreness that soon yields to relief and greater mobility.

Scar Tissue Mobilization

Any patient who has had abdominal or pelvic surgery will have scar tissue, and the inflammation of endo's implants can also cause scar-like material to build up. In both cases, the scarring restricts movement, but it is a normal and healthy part of healing; scar tissue is the all-purpose repair material of the body. No, it does not possess the same qualities as the original tissue, but it is moldable and pliable and can be made to perform just like the tissue you were born with.

Of course, there's a catch: If you wait too long, the scars may adhere to the surrounding tissue or organ or nerve, and that is not healthy. It is why orthopedic surgeons now almost routinely recommend PT four to six weeks after surgery, and it is why women with endo also need a PT intervention.

Scar tissue mobilization, which constitutes that intervention, is exactly what its name implies. That is because scar tissue, both visible and invisible, tightens and shortens the muscles and fascia, creating tension and restricting movement—up to and including the point of spasm—thus contributing substantively to the patient's pelvic and abdominal pain. Working mostly externally but in some cases internally as well, the physical therapist mobilizes even the unseen scars that endometriosis or any possible surgery may have caused. The technique is in effect a massage of the area, which releases the scar tissue, helping to improve elasticity and flexibility and loosening tissue-on-tissue adherence.

Neural Mobilization

The axon of a nerve is the long, threadlike fiber that serves as a pathway for impulses that stimulate or inhibit an action—often a sensory perception like feeling hot or cold, but also actions affecting muscles and organs. So maintaining the efficiency of those pathways is essential to keeping the nervous system humming and muscles and organs functioning at peak performance. Fascial tissue damage caused by endo implants that stretch and pull nerves threatens that efficiency; it disrupts the nerve flow and slows axonal transport. The technique of neural mobilization is a form of gentle palpation that helps free any restrictions on the nerve flow, gets the nerves sliding and gliding again, and thereby optimizes and speeds up that axonal transport.

Visceral Mobilization

Organs need to move in order to execute their essential functions. The bladder must expand and contract sufficiently to fill up and empty out. The bowel needs "give" so it won't restrict the natural passage of stool. The uterus needs to expand to accommodate a growing fetus. **BOTTOM LINE:** When organs don't move well, neither do you. So while fascia and muscles must hold organs in place, motion is a requirement.

And endo can undermine this needed organ motion. The inflammation it causes through its painful scarring and restricting eventually makes organs adhere to one another, which in turn distorts what's inside the pelvic cavity, pulling on the underlying muscles and stressing the attachment of those muscles and fascia to the bones. End result: restricted motion, with consequences.

For example, if your rectum is restricted due to endometriosis implants on the uterosacral ligaments—a common place for endo to show up—the rectum will neither fill nor empty sufficiently. It simply will be unable to do what it is built to do, which is to enable the efficient passing of feces. It's why constipation is so common among endo sufferers.

Moreover, these same endo restrictions in the pelvis may also affect joints and bony structures. For example, endo-generated distortions in the pelvis may prevent the normal physiological movement of the sacrum, thereby increasing tension in the muscles attaching to and around the sacrum. If the sacrum and its muscles don't move well, you don't either—and you probably suffer back pain into the bargain.

What a qualified physical therapist can do that is so valuable to endo sufferers is to apply gentle but very targeted manual techniques to mobilize each of the organs in turn, working through the ligaments, muscles, or fascia that support the organs and keep them in place. How do they do it?

"We use the organs as handles," says Corey Hazama, one of the most highly skilled pelvic-health visceral manipulation therapists in the United States. "We localize the restriction as specifically as possible, then mobilize either into the direction the organ 'wants' us to go or toward the greatest barrier point of the restriction till we create the release and restore mobility."*

---

* Hazama attributes her skills in palpation—knowing what a restriction feels like and how to release it—to her training in Functional Manual Therapy™ taught by the Institute of Physical Art and to Jean-Pierre Barral of the Barral Institute.

That restoration of mobility releases the blood and other fluids so they can flow freely again. The renewed movements put the brain on alert that the organs are ready to function, and that helps down-regulate the nervous system. If slowly moving organs are the primary contributor to an endo patient's pain—not to mention that their sluggishness makes the body function inefficiently—visceral mobilization is an essential early treatment due to the hierarchy of protection in the body—i.e., organs are what the body most wants to protect.

Joint Mobilization

We can't forget the joints. After all, we need them to move. The sacrum won't move, for example, unless the sacroiliac joint moves it. Ditto for the hip joint and spine, which have also been known to refer organ-like pain to the abdomino-pelvic region. Since we know that endo's reach through the musculoskeletal system can be almost limitless, it's therefore essential to make sure all joints move optimally.

All of these manual therapies can be carried out both internally and externally and may need to be performed both vaginally and rectally in order to ensure that *all* the pain is addressed. Obviously, the internal techniques may be done only with patient consent and to patient tolerance. All such treatments should be performed in a private treatment room, and a chaperone may be requested if the patient is a minor or would simply feel more comfortable with another person present. Amy says there are few things more gratifying than releasing an endo sufferer's muscular trigger point, internally or externally, and hearing her exclamation of recognition: "That's it! That's my pain! And it's gone!" But it is a moment every patient deserves to experience in a safe and private environment.

NEUROMUSCULAR REEDUCATION

You can't ask a patient to sit up straight if her muscles are so short that sitting up straight is painful. It is not unusual to find endo sufferers who spend so much time curled up in a ball as a response to their menstrual pain, clenching their abdominal and pelvic muscles, that the muscles have adapted and have shortened over time out of habit—while their back muscles, as a result, have grown weak.

There's more. Muscles that hold the pelvic floor in place have tightened up, and everything that goes on in the pelvic floor has probably gone amiss—bladder, bowel, and sexual function. Moreover, these tightened muscles limit joint mobility. They undermine muscle tone. Overall, they adversely affect the woman's posture and movement. Before anything else can happen in the way of remedy, those muscles need to be reeducated to their "proper" length and tension and must be retaught when to contract and when to relax so that the muscles have the endurance to meet your body's demands.

Luckily, there is a range of physical therapy techniques that can help return such patients to the point where they can sit up straight. One likely technique is *proprioceptive neuromuscular facilitation* (PNF).[9] Originally devised as a rehabilitation methodology for patients with such neuromuscular diagnoses as Parkinson's and multiple sclerosis, PNF focuses on stretching and contracting the muscles as a way to increase flexibility and restore them to their proper length. In this technique, a physical therapist activates the patient's proprioceptors—the body's internal gyroscope-like positioning sensors—to provide the motor information for the patient to initiate a particular movement or posture by a single body part or group of body parts.

Here's how it works: The therapist wants to excite certain inactive muscles and tone down muscles that have been working too hard. To do this, the therapist cues the patient on how and what to move, exciting the proprioceptive sensors in the inactive muscles and calming the sensors in the overworked muscles—thus also affecting the relevant tendons, bones, and joints. The goal is balance, an attempt to put an end to compensating movements that guard against pain.

Obviously, this is not something you want to do on your own. (There is also a version of PNF intended for developing athletic prowess, not for rehabilitation, but that is not what we are referring to here.) A physical therapist trained in the technique will steer you clear of potential injuries to tendons, muscles, ligaments, etc., and will target the right muscle groups to be reeducated. Done correctly, PNF can be very helpful in returning these muscles to their true length so they won't clench again. And that, in turn, can alleviate pain and tension.

One of the more common techniques of PNF is the *contract-relax stretch*. Basically, what you do is contract the muscle being targeted. For example, if it is the hamstring, you would contract the muscle, then stretch it. The lengthening relaxes the muscle and extends range of motion. Contract-relax is a type of isotonic stretch that is a more advanced form of flexibility training than plain old stretching.

Another very straightforward example of neuromuscular reeducation is teaching the patient proper posture and body mechanics. These can be relearned, even after faulty postures and mechanics have resulted in dysfunction, and new behaviors can be made habitual. We often see endo patients with pelvic pain sitting on just one side of the sit bone, often with legs flexed and crossed and likely with pelvic misalignment. Such postures increase joint stress. They shorten the muscles on one side only, thus producing the imbalances that form trigger points and tissue restrictions and thereby ignite abdomino-pelvic pain. Again, a physical therapist appropriately trained in the musculoskeletal system can determine the right reeducation or corrective measures.

Such measures may include strategies on how best to empty your bowels and bladder without straining or feeling the need to push, learning instead to lose the tension and coordinate your abdominal muscles so you can evacuate comfortably and completely. Similarly, we educate patients in sexual function, proper postures or positioning, and how to relax. More on all these strategies in chapters 4, 5, and 6.

Biofeedback,* via a specialized machine, using a mirror or a finger, or simply with verbal cueing, is another important aid to the neuromuscular reeducation of the pelvic floor. When a patient can see or be instantly "notified" that she has tightened a muscle or suffered a spasm in her pelvic floor, she can make the connection between the symptom that bothers her and the trigger that caused it. When the therapist then calms the tightening and directs the patient to lengthen the muscles, the biofeedback on that action reinforces clarity. The relief the patient feels becomes a springboard for repeating the cause-and-effect lesson, with the patient releasing more tension and lengthening the muscles further each time.

THERAPEUTIC EXERCISE: THE BASIC SIX

Part of the physical therapy treatment for endo is learning specific movements that you can practice on your own at home. Keep in

---

* One caution here: Biofeedback should be a supervised modality and an added resource, not a sole solution. In other words, if a patient is left alone in the room to do biofeedback as the sole modality of her physical therapy, she should find another physical therapist.

mind that these movements are only accompaniments to what you do with your PT—your physical therapist—in the office. And keep in mind also that if you've had endo symptoms for some years, your muscles have been tight for a long time—and that cannot be undone by just performing a few exercises a few times in the bedroom. As we have emphasized, there is no quick fix.

But in Amy's experience, six basic exercises get you started. They gently stretch the muscles and of course stimulate the cardiovascular system; getting you moving is essential to any healing process. All of these actions may help release the tension in the musculoskeletal system and cool the central nervous system—equally essential to your healing. But note: Not all of these exercises work for all people.

Still, these six very simple therapeutic exercises are basic and therefore a start to beating the muscle tightening of endo. We call them the Basic Six, and they will reappear as recommendations throughout this book. Aimed at loosening the tightness in your abdomino-pelvic area and, by extension, throughout the body, the Basic Six are a great way to start the day, every day. Moreover, you can do some of them just about anywhere, so please do, and however you can manage it, try to do them more than once a day. Remember to start small and easily—no overexertion, no exhausting yourself. If you cannot do the stated number of repetitions or hold the stretch or position for very long at first, don't push it; you will get there eventually. It took a long time for your abdomino-pelvic area to become this tense and painful, and you cannot change that overnight. But this is the way to begin.

Exercise 1: Breathe

This is conscious breathing—slow and deep. Inhale from deep down, and as you breathe in, visualize the air expanding your belly outward and your ribs to the sides as you let your pelvic floor "open" till the air fills your lungs. Take from three to five seconds for the inhalation. Pause one second. Then, keeping the pelvic floor open, exhale for even longer—five or six seconds—from the top down, letting the air flow out of your lungs, then relaxing your ribs and belly.

Pause one second. Repeat. Do five repetitions.

Exercise 2: Pelvic Floor Drop

The pelvic floor drop copies the sensation of relief you feel when you urinate—in particular, the sort of blanket of relaxation you feel when the need to urinate has been delayed and has become somewhat urgent and you are finally able to let go. This is therefore an exercise that is as much mental as physical; it is your brain and a very subtle motion of release by the muscles that go to work here. You can do this exercise while standing, walking, sitting, lying down, stretching—whatever is comfortable for you.

Start by relaxing your body and closing your eyes. Breathe in consciously and deeply, as in Exercise 1. With the inhale, let go of your pelvic muscles—just drop them—and with the exhale, visualize the air flowing out of your body, and maintain the drop.

Do the pelvic floor drop with deep breathing first thing in the morning, twice an hour throughout the day if you can, during any exercise, and whenever you feel any pelvic pain or increased bladder or bowel urgency or frequency—sexual pain too. In fact, if and when you feel tension in any part of your body, this exercise can help release it.

Exercise 3: Pelvic Floor Stretch

You can do this stretch squatting or lying down, whichever is possible or easiest for you. If you have hip, knee, or back pain or dysfunction, do it only in the lying-down position.

If you are able to squat, stand with your legs apart, feet extending a few inches beyond the shoulders, toes turned slightly outward, and, keeping your back as straight as possible, squat down till your rear is six to eight inches off the floor; use a wall for support if you need to. Relax into the position, arms resting inside your thighs, hands together or relaxed to the floor, as you breathe from six to eight deep breaths and drop the pelvic floor. Again keeping your back straight, place your hands on your knees and push yourself up.

If you do the stretch lying down, lie on your back on a firm surface, and bring your knees up to your chest and the soles of your feet together. Use your hands to hold your knees flared outward in whatever way is comfortable for you. Stretch the position gradually and progressively for six to eight deep breaths as you drop the pelvic floor. Do not bounce, and do not push hard.

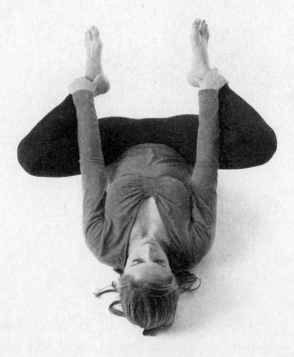

Do two to three repetitions twice a day.

4. Hip Rotator Stretch

Here is a gentle, steady stretch to loosen the muscles you use to rotate and turn at the hip—muscles that, when tightened, limit your ability to make those moves *and* stress your pelvic floor. Lie on your back, with both knees bent and your head resting on a thin pillow. Raise your right knee and rest your right ankle on your left thigh in a figure-four position. Now lift your left leg and wrap both your hands around the back of your left thigh. Pull the left thigh gently toward you; you should feel the stretch in your right buttock and possibly around the hip. Hold the stretch for six to eight deep breaths.

Switch: left ankle on right thigh, right leg raised, pull right thigh toward you, hold, feel the stretch in your left buttock and hip region.

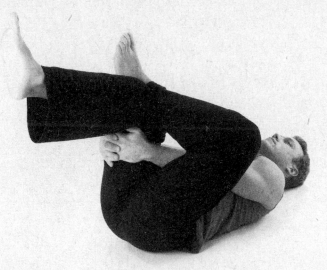

Do two to four repetitions per day.

5. Hip Flexor Stretch

The flexors are the muscles that let you lift your thigh, bend, and—obviously—flex, so when they are under tension, your mobility suffers. Here's how to stretch these muscles:

Stand straight with feet hip-width apart. Step forward two to three feet, if you can, with your right foot. Obviously, the length of your forward movement will be determined by your height and thus the length of your stride, or by the tightness of your muscles. Balancing by holding on to the top of a chair or sofa, keep your pelvis square and bend your right knee into a lunge position. Don't let the right knee extend out over the toes. Feel the stretch in the front of the *left* thigh and hip region, and if you don't, keep the pelvis square and lunge farther forward. Hold the stretch for six to eight deep breaths, then switch: step forward with the left foot, bend the left knee into a lunge, feel the stretch along the front of the *right* thigh.

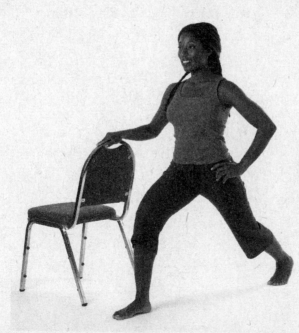

Do two to four repetitions per day.

6. Abdominal Stretch

This stretch is aimed at lengthening the abdominal muscles just above the pelvic floor. Lie flat on your stomach on a mat or blanket and bring your hands up next to your shoulders, palms down flat. If that position is uncomfortable, rest on your elbows instead. Inhale deeply, as instructed in Exercise 1, and as you exhale, push your upper body up slowly with both hands as your hips and legs remain flat and relaxed. Straighten your arms as much as possible. Hold for six to eight deep breaths.

If it's hard for you to straighten your arms, or if you have shoulder, wrist, or elbow problems, you can do this standing upright. Feet should be hip-width apart with knees slightly bent. Place your hands on either side of your lower back, just at the top of the butt. Inhale deeply as in Exercise 1. Exhale, slowly bending your torso backward until you feel a gentle stretch in your abdominal muscles and the upper part of your thighs. Hold for two to four deep breaths.

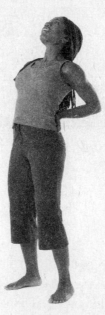

Do two to four repetitions a day either way.

Any and all of these therapeutic exercises will stimulate the cardiovascular system as well as stretch and loosen your muscles, and few things are as essential to healing and to feeling better as movement that gets the blood flowing and keeps it flowing. That is why it is important, in addition to these six exercises (and others in this book), simply to get up and get moving. One caveat: If you recently had surgery or if your pain increases at all as you begin to move, do be sure to obtain the approval of your doctor or PT for when to start and how much to do.

Yes, we do know how hard getting up and getting moving can be for women debilitated by their pain. We have seen patients who literally could not walk across the room without pain, others who were unable to get out of bed. But there is really only one way to get up and get moving, and that is to get up, then move. A few steps constitute a beginning. Wait a few hours, then do the same few steps again. Do them another few hours later and again a few hours after that. Even two or three times a day, even for three minutes each time, will help. Every day that you get up and move is a day closer to regaining your life.

And if you are able, the simplest as well as one of the best cardiovascular exercises is walking. Not walking as a means to a destination but walking as exercise. Not as furious exercise either. Rather, the intent should be a brisk but comfortable pace that is steadily maintained. Iris adds: Leave your phone at home; enjoy this walk for its own sake. Start with five minutes—twice a day. Work your way up from there. A particularly effective walking exercise is doing it in a body of water. You're expending healthy effort against the water, but because of the buoyancy, there is little stress on the joints.

Whatever form of exercise you choose, make it something you enjoy—but not something that is too high-intensity. You're not out to kill it, nor to stir up buckets of sweat. If the point of the exercise is to squeeze your core or tuck your "tush" or if the activity exacerbates any of your symptoms, find another form of exercise. A good idea is to ask your physical therapist which exercise of those you enjoy is actually going to benefit what you and the PT are trying to achieve in therapy. Look on it as an investment in yourself—in your health—and therefore as quality time just for you, away from the computer, the job, the family. Don't think of "fitness" as your aim and don't measure yourself against others. Remember how good it felt when you were in command of a strong, capable body? Your real goal is to recapture that feeling—and then to keep at it.

TREATMENT MODALITIES

The manual therapies, musculoskeletal and neuromuscular reeducation, and therapeutic exercise that a patient can do on her own are not the end of physical therapy's treatment capabilities. The physical therapist's manual skills are augmented with a range of what the profession calls "modalities" used to decrease pain wherever it occurs, lessen inflammation in the top layer of tissue, and help relax muscles. Amy cautions that these modalities are adjuncts only; they do not substitute for the PT treatments we've just outlined. But they can be helpful in certain cases. Here is a brief overview of these additional treatments.

Low-level or "cold" laser therapy emits photon light without heat and provides stimulation at the cellular level. This handheld modality can assist in relieving trigger points, alleviating minor muscle and joint aches, lessening pain, reducing stiffness, breaking up a muscle spasm or scar adhesion, and increasing lymph flow.

Therapeutic ultrasound uses a transducer to produce low-intensity, low-frequency sound waves that warm and stimulate the tissues of a highly targeted, very small area. Practically speaking, it is used most commonly to relieve pain in the perineal body—the area between the vaginal opening and the anal-rectal opening. It can help increase the flow of blood and oxygen to the affected area— typically, connective tissue, ligaments, tendons, fascia, and scar tissue. Again, the effect is to decrease pain, which is why ultrasound, along with manual therapy, is typically recommended as effective for patients who suffer the pain of penetration during sexual intercourse.

Electrical stimulation can help relax muscle spasms, increase blood flow, and may result in increased range of motion in the tissues and in reeducation of the muscles. But for some portion of the patient population, the internal device, aimed at interrupting the electrical currents of pain signals and thereby limiting the number of signals that reach the brain, can actually be more aggravating than useful. Amy's experience with the device is that more than half of pain patients feel worse after undergoing treatment.

Transcutaneous electrical nerve stimulation (TENS) applies mild electrical stimulation via electrodes on or near the pain to reduce its impact. It is based on a principle called gate control theory— the idea that non-painful input closes the gates on painful input. This modality works externally and often superficially, and while it is effective for some women in alleviating symptoms, for others it offers little relief.

Applied heat and cold are classic modalities of temporary pain relief. Heat, applied as often as you want, relaxes tense muscles and spurs blood flow. Cold, applied for twenty minutes three to four times a day, constricts the blood vessels where the cold is applied and helps to decrease inflammation and thus pain. Heating pads and ice packs will do just fine; be sure to protect the skin with a thin towel.

All these modalities are rightly part of the toolkit of a skilled physical therapist and may be applied as recommended.

HOW LONG WILL IT TAKE?

Undertaking physical therapy is a commitment. Most sessions that address abdominal and pelvic floor pain last one hour, and sessions are preferably held on a weekly or twice-weekly basis. Although it typically takes months to feel substantially better—and of course individual cases differ—patients typically experience some improvement within the first four weeks, definitely by eight weeks. Such improvement is an indication that you are on the right track.

Here are two basic cautions to keep in mind as you begin your PT.

1. Don't be surprised if you experience new kinds of pain at first; it means that the muscles and tissue are getting reeducated, and the new soreness will fade in time, especially as your therapist becomes more familiar with your body. Muscles, joints, tendons, and fascia that have been "locked" and inflamed for a long period of time do not easily or quickly unravel, cool down, and return to form. They are stubborn in that respect. But as Amy told Elena back in chapter 2, pain at the outset can be a signal that your central nervous system is responding to what's happening; that means the therapy is working, and that means you want to keep at it. Also, be assured it's temporary—lasting no more than a couple of days.

2. Mental stress causes the same reactions in the body as does physical stress, and being mentally stressed while trying to heal is a barrier to achieving what you're trying to achieve.

It's hard, of course, not to bring that stress with you to the PT session or to your at-home therapeutic exercises. But try, if you can, to leave it behind. Practice your deep breathing throughout the day, and try practicing ten to fifteen minutes of meditation twice a day, as we'll discuss in greater detail in chapter 10. We've seen what happens when patients let their stress get the better of them: Either they tend to become inconsistent in doing the therapy—they do it "sort of," or halfway, or just skip sessions—or they decide that their progress isn't dramatic enough and become disillusioned. Both the inconsistency and the disillusionment exacerbate the stress and slow the progress even further.

You *will* feel the difference; it will take time.

Paying for the Physical Therapy You Need

Yes, physical therapy at the level we are recommending is a highly skilled practice, and whatever your insurance plan, there are likely to be out-of-pocket expenses in the form of co-pays, deductibles, co-insurance, or fees for service. You will want to look carefully at your own plan, check with your Human Resources department at work, and confer with the doctor prescribing your PT to try to work out a process that makes sense for you.

But what's the definition of "making sense"?

Patients sometimes complain to Iris that they cannot afford the PT she prescribes now; they would rather put it off to a later date. She'll then ask them to consider that delaying what you need now to a later date really means you will need more therapy at that time—and probably more complicated and demanding therapy as well. That also means that it will take longer for you to get better. Obviously, more therapy over a longer period of time will cost even more. In other words, what could be eight weeks of PT if you start today might be four months of PT if you don't start till after you've paid off your car loan or till "after the holidays" or till spring arrives.

At bottom, it is a question of priorities. Supplementing your insurance coverage or paying a therapist directly right now may seem pricey, but weigh it against your suffering and your health before you decide you cannot afford it.

ENDO AND THE BLADDER

Resting on the pelvic floor and located in front of the uterus, the bladder is a hollow organ made of smooth but elastic muscle that acts as a temporary storage depot for the urine made by your kidneys.

Your kidneys filter fluid, derived from both drinking and eating, at a rate of about 120 ounces every minute, although far less than a teaspoon of those 120 fluid ounces becomes urine. The urine, quite simply, is what remains once the kidneys have refined out the waste and excess water from the fluid. Two long connecting tubes called ureters, one from each kidney, transport the urine to openings in the bladder. These openings are one-way valves, so there's no backflow.

When empty, the bladder is about 2³/₄ inches long—as is traditionally said, about the size of a pear—but it stretches as it fills, distending to as much as nearly twice that size. It typically takes somewhere between 10 and 17 fluid ounces before nerves start sending you the feeling that you want to empty the bladder—although the bladder can hold considerably more than that, despite the urge. Your bladder muscle involuntarily contracts, and the voiding happens through a tiny exit hole at the bottom of the bladder, the urethra. You relax your sphincter, which otherwise "guards" the urethra, and the urine flows.

The process, engineered over the eons by evolution, is thus a fairly simple one and very effective—until or unless one or more of any number of triggers begins to generate dysfunctions, discomfort, and pain.

The effects of all this might begin when you notice that you are urinating more frequently than you used to. You feel like you have emptied your bladder, yet just moments later—or so it seems—you feel the need to empty it again.

You find yourself checking out the location of the nearest toilet whenever you leave home. As if that weren't annoying enough, maybe you experience an occasional burning sensation when you urinate and sometimes pain or pressure in the bladder even when you don't. And since, as we've noted repeatedly, the symptoms you present with tend to determine which specialist you go to, the typical next step is an appointment with a urologist.

Historically, after running the usual test for bacteria and infection, the symptoms we've just noted will prompt the urologist to perform a test to gauge how much the bladder can hold and then assess the bladder's dynamics—typically by asking the patient to keep a diary of the liquid she drinks, noting what it is and when and how much of it she takes in, and when and how often she voids. The likely diagnosis of these symptoms will be interstitial cystitis—IC—officially defined by the Interstitial Cystitis Association as "a bladder condition" with "multiple symptoms" that may include pelvic pain, pressure or discomfort in the bladder and in the pelvic region, plus urinary frequency and/or urgency. It is what the profession calls a diagnosis of exclusion—arrived at once you have ruled out everything else.

The connective tissue that makes up the interior coating of the bladder is composed of glycosaminoglycans, which serve as lubricants and thus enable this interior coating to protect the bladder. Scientists refer to these glycosaminoglycans as GAGs, which is why the interior coating of the bladder that they compose is called the GAG layer. Any malfunction of the GAG layer—any gaps or leaks in its surface, for example—can start a chain of painful and unpleasant reactions. In a typical case, toxins or irritants from certain foods pass through the gaps in the tissue and prompt mast cells to release histamines, just as in an allergic reaction. In fact, many women diagnosed with IC tend to have several other kinds of allergies, and allergic susceptibility typically exists alongside IC.

A common urological answer to these IC symptoms is a very minimal dose of medication that doubles as a treatment for anxiety or depression and that can moderate the sensation of urgency significantly. But in a great many cases, the relief is temporary, which is why so many women become ensnared in a cycle of return visits to the urologist and increasingly complex treatments: more or more powerful medications, and possibly a procedure known as bladder instillation—in which a small catheter is inserted into the bladder where it ejects a "cocktail" of medicines to help heal the bladder from the inside; the patient eventually expels these through urination.

Instillations tend to work well—if IC is the only issue. But there is a compelling reason why so many of these standard IC treatments may fail to "solve" the issue. It is that all of the symptoms of bladder pain and dysfunction that prompt the treatments can also be related to endometriosis or musculoskeletal issues—either directly or as a downstream result of the process of cell growth and expansion. Moreover, these standard treatments tend to be used in isolation, and they should be used in conjunction with proper endo treatment. So while some of the IC tools a urologist prescribes to relieve the symptoms may help briefly, those patients for whom unsuspected and undiagnosed endo is the first cause of the symptoms will always be playing catch-up with the pain and dysfunction. *Their* pain and dysfunction, after all, spring from a source somewhat different from the one for which they are being treated—and are also fundamentally chronic.

As long ago as 2002, a group of doctors and medical researchers led by Dr. Maurice K. Chung, a renowned surgeon and expert in the field of female pelvic medicine,* published a study entitled "The Evil Twins of Chronic Pelvic Pain Syndrome: Endometriosis and Interstitial Cystitis."[10] The study found that more than 90 percent of women with confirmed endo also had the symptoms routinely diagnosed as IC. That's what makes the two diseases "evil twins": The symptoms traditionally labeled as endometriosis can be identical to those of interstitial cystitis—and vice versa.

What is particularly frustrating about this pairing of disease processes is that even decades after the Chung study, the medical community hasn't quite caught up with its findings—although as we write this, there is encouraging evidence that more and more doctors and other practitioners are beginning to parse the IC label more carefully. The belief that IC is the single underlying cause of a chain of pain and dysfunctions is less widely held than it once was, and there is a growing recognition that the use of the term as a catchall for the pain and dysfunctions is no longer adequate.

---

* Currently president at Ohio's Midwest Regional Center of Excellence for Endometriosis, Pelvic Pain & Female Pelvic Medicine.

Medically, that is critical, because if you diagnose endo-related bladder dysfunction as IC and treat it solely with IC tools, you are addressing only part of the problem—just one of the evil twins. And since we cited back in chapter 1 that half the women with endo suffer the symptoms of what is called interstitial cystitis, that is a lot of suffering women for whom IC tools alone won't be enough.

There's yet another reason they won't be enough. It isn't just that the traditionally accepted symptoms of IC are virtually identical to the traditionally accepted symptoms of endo; so are the traditionally accepted symptoms of musculoskeletal dysfunction in the abdomino-pelvic region. Interstitial cystitis, endometriosis, and musculoskeletal dysfunction are triplets; if not exactly identical triplets, they are surely related. And women who suffer those musculoskeletal symptoms of the "third" triplet—the varied aches and pains, the structural misalignments, the bladder and bowel disorders, the sexual dysfunction and more—are just as likely to be treated with the same limited IC tools as women with bladder "issues" and women with endo. Such treatment is unlikely to be enough to bring relief or to affect the underlying cause.

In fact, most medical practitioners no longer use the term *interstitial cystitis*. Even the website of the Interstitial Cystitis Association at www.ichelp.org now confirms that "IC is also referred to as painful bladder syndrome, bladder pain syndrome, and hypersensitive bladder syndrome," the latter a term nobody uses. The key is in the word *syndrome*, an acknowledgment that there are a bunch of associated symptoms causing a variety of pain and dysfunction around the term IC. The medley of titles for that pain and dysfunction reflects the continuing uncertainty over the ground rules for diagnosis and is evidence of the confusion surrounding both the causes and the effects of what is going on in the pelvic region in general and in the urinary tract in particular. To us, it makes sense to wrap it all in the blanket term known as painful bladder syndrome (PBS).

But whatever you call it, it can be debilitating.

THE ENDO TRIGGER

As we've noted before, for most but not all women, pain is the primary defining symptom of endometriosis, and menstrual cramps can be a common form of that pain. Every girl or woman who has felt such cramps knows well how the pain impels you to tense the muscles within the pelvis. That not only amplifies the pain further, it also affects the bladder in ways that can lead to urinary dysfunction.

Urogynecologist Dr. Charles Butrick has long studied the ways endo can affect the bladder, and he has a lot to say on the subject:

"The severity and duration of these menstrual cramps can result in two major changes within the pelvis. The first change is that because of this pain, patients will often tense their muscles to the point that the muscles become a new source of pain and dysfunction. When the pelvic floor muscles tighten, it not only results in a feeling of pressure and discomfort coming from the muscles but often will result in problems of urinary hesitancy and difficulty passing urine. This quickly results in . . . urinary frequency, bladder pain syndromes, and at times bladder infections.

"The second major change is that when patients have pain that goes on for many months, often the nerves in the pelvis become hypersensitive. Those same nerves make the bladder hypersensitive; therefore when the patient has two ounces in her bladder it will sometimes feel like twenty. This of course results in symptoms of urinary frequency and bladder pain. These symptoms are the classic findings described in painful bladder syndrome; the old term was *interstitial cystitis*."

Old term or new, IC or PBS or musculoskeletal dysfunction, to anyone who has suffered its symptoms, the terminology is beside the point. The routine sensation that you have 20 ounces of urine pressing down on your bladder, or, maybe just as bad, the fear that you are going to have that sensation all day long, can limit your lifestyle and add to your stress. If you are "going" a few times an hour or even hourly, are hesitant to leave your house, are nervous about getting on a train or bus, dread the idea of a meeting at work, or feel you need to make special arrangements if you go to a movie or the theater, that equates to tight boundaries on how you live. Add in the pain, and the misery quotient rises even further.

Limits on Women's Lives, in Patients' Words:

"I get up at night anywhere from two to six times to urinate..."

"At times, it hurts to urinate..."

"I pee fifteen to twenty times a day..."

"I pee eight to ten times an hour..."

"I'm the one we stop for on car trips—time and time again..."

"I have to push my urine out..."

"My friends always tell me I have a small bladder..."

"I never fully empty my bladder..."

"My urinary symptoms are worse during my period..."

"I urinate five times before I go to bed to try to empty my bladder..."

"After I pee, I always feel I have to pee again..."

"I always feel like I have a urinary tract infection..."

"It burns when I urinate..."

It is totally understandable that women whose lives are limited by one or more of these boundaries see the problem as a urinary issue, a bladder issue, and are motivated to see a urologist. If you are racing to the ladies' room every fifteen minutes in an eight-hour work day, you're not thinking "gynecological" or "musculo-skeletal"; you're focused on how to stop this exhaustingly frequent urination. Thus begins the typical series of urological treatments to relieve this and other symptoms—all too often with minimal effectiveness and temporarily only.

Iris estimates that seven out of ten of her endo patients have concomitant painful bladder syndrome but were never properly di-agnosed despite complaints of urinary frequency, urinary urgency, and "bladder pain" before being referred to her. Amy says five out of ten of her patients have been diagnosed with PBS. Over the course of their urological treatments, these patients have "tried ev-erything"—a range of medications, bladder instillations, in some cases bladder surgery—but nothing worked, or it worked only tem-porarily. In other words, the treatments can work, but they work best when all of a woman's symptoms have been identified and are being treated comprehensively.

If you search for a urologist on what we both refer to as "Dr. Google," and if you're in pain and discomfort, you may not notice that the urologist nearest you actually specializes in pros-tate cases. This is a specialist unlikely to have expert knowledge of endometriosis. He is also unlikely to know much about pelvic floor muscle dysfunction, which is not much of a bread-and-butter issue in his urological specialty. So this urologist's treatments for your pain and discomfort will certainly be incomplete. Against the many hands on a stove that the panoply of symptoms both endo and PBS can represent—not just urinary frequency but the tensed muscles, the impact on skeletal structure, pain throughout the pelvic area, nerves igniting an upregulated central nervous system—medications to relax the bladder are going to have minimal effect. A fuller picture is required.

SEEING THE FULL PICTURE

On the other hand, patients who consult Iris for what they assume is a *gynecological* issue or Amy for what they figure is a *musculoskeletal* or *pelvic floor* issue might wonder why they are being asked to fill out a form and answer questions about their urinary frequency and urgency. The form, known as the PUF (Pain, Urgency, Frequency) questionnaire, scores the number of times the patient voids during the day and how often she gets up at night to do so—and much more. Both of us, in our initial one-on-one consultations with patients, press the point further and ask a number of questions to get to the core issues. Do they hit the ladies' room more frequently than their coworkers? Are they known as the "small-bladder person" in the carpool? If the patient's spouse or partner has come with her and is in the room, we solicit that observer's take on how many times the patient *really* gets up to pee at night *before* falling asleep—as well as after.

We'll ask patients if they've ever had a UTI—urinary tract infection—and for the seven out of ten of Iris's patients and the five out of ten of Amy's already diagnosed with PBS/IC, more often than not, the answer will be "several, but the cultures were negative," yet the patient was nevertheless prescribed antibiotics.

We ask how much coffee and tea the patient drinks, whether she likes spicy foods, if she drinks carbonated beverages—all of them items that tend to irritate the bladders of women with PBS/IC. Patients who pride themselves on their fitness and who spend time at the gym or in yoga class will boast of their preference for bottled electrolyte waters—perhaps not realizing that ingredients in these beverages typically include substances like acids and potassium that can severely irritate a troubled bladder.

Almost always, we find, we need to work hard to tease the information out of patients. After all, they have come to consult a gynecologist about painful periods or painful intercourse, or to have a physical therapist manipulate away their abdominal and pelvic pain. They can't figure out why either of us is asking them about their bladder.

The answer of course is that the disease processes of endo, PBS, and musculoskeletal dysfunction all require their own multidimensional approach. It is necessary to know which dimensions of a patient's discomfort and dysfunction have been identified and treated, what has helped them and what has not helped, not just how many hands are touching a hot stove but what those hands are. Thus informed, we can begin the physical examination that lets us understand just where and how to begin treating the individual.

Further evidence of the uncertainties and discord over bladder pain and endo's effect on it is that the two of us sort of disagree on what painful bladder syndrome is all about. *Sort* of. We are of one mind that the syndrome's multiple symptoms arise from a combination of an upregulated central nervous system, distortions of the pelvic anatomy and thus of the muscles and fascia of the pelvis, and the immune system's mast cells releasing histamines from the lining of the bladder—histamines that in turn increase food and environmental sensitivities. And we agree emphatically that endo can be the first cause of all these impacts.

Our difference of opinion—more a difference of outlook or emphasis—not too surprisingly reflects our professional biases.

For Iris, PBS is a particular pathology with its own progression within the individual patient. The progression will be unique to the individual but will affect and be affected by the upregulated central nervous system, the musculoskeletal distortions, and the immune system firing up inflammation.

She has seen and excised endo implants from the walls of women's bladders, and she has observed how endo implants may affect the nearby anatomy of fascia, muscle, organs, and bones and up-regulate the spinal segment above and below which the bladder* is specifically stimulated. This amplifies pain, increases inflammatory responses, and releases histamines that generate whole new categories of pain.

In Amy's view, the primary driver of the PBS sufferer's pain is most often musculoskeletal. The anatomical distortions from the endo implants cause mechanical dysfunction and generate viscero-somatic/somatic-visceral cross-talk. So, for example, the pain originally caused by implants that affect the uterus or rectum "talks" viscero-somatically to the abdominal muscles, causing them to become irritated, and those muscles then somato-viscerally talk to and aggravate the bladder or the nerves that assist in bladder function.

As she explains, this is why bladder pain can sometimes make you feel, among other things, that you can find relief by urinating. Over time, the mind reflexively conflates the irritation with the need to urinate, and to avoid such frequent urination, you tighten your pelvic floor muscles even further, and those tightened muscles in turn irritate the organ yet more and propel even more frequency. From organ to body and from body to organ, the cycle simply escalates as cross-talk amplifies the inflammation both ways.

---

* The bowel too, as we'll see in chapter 5.

Amy also points out that it is possible for both men and women to suffer the discomfort and dysfunction of PBS without having the gaps in the interstitium of the bladder that often characterize PBS and without having endo; in her practice, some 35 percent of PBS patients are male. And she notes also that a number of her otherwise healthy PT patients grew up being told repeatedly to urinate before leaving home, or were advised to avoid public toilets, or were urged by parents to "hold it in"—all with deleterious musculoskeletal consequences.

But if we disagree in part on what constitutes PBS, we are in accord on how to address its impact: For just about every patient suffering from painful bladder syndrome, PT and dietary changes are central. Mostly, the two work effectively together. But there are those patients for whom either dietary change or PT on its own does the trick of reducing the inflammation and thus calming the system. And, as Amy often cautions, there are some people for whom the particular limitations of a diet aimed at easing the bladder can adversely affect the gastrointestinal system. If that is the case—that is, if certain foods tend to aggravate your GI system—modify the diet and continue on the PT.

CHANGING YOUR DIET

The aim of the dietary approach is to identify those foods, if any, that may be aggravating your painful bladder syndrome so as to eliminate them from your diet or at least reduce your intake. This is a food avoidance diet; it is not aimed at weight loss but at steering clear of certain foods and not others. The foods to steer clear of are those with a high content of acids and potassium, which, where the bladder is concerned, constitute high-aggravation substances. What's the best way to do this? We have a recommendation, and it's this:

Reproduce and then follow this link—https://ic-network.com /downloads/2012icnfoodlist.pdf. It is the 2012 IC Network food list, divided into three categories, Usually Bladder Friendly, Foods Worth Trying, and Foods to Avoid. Caution: This list is *not* an anti-inflammatory list; it only references acids and potassium, so temper your diet changes with what you know about pro- and anti-inflammatory. For example, lard is in the Usually Bladder-Friendly column, but don't start eating lard. With that caution in mind, here's how Iris says to proceed:

For a minimum of eight weeks, eat only what's in the left-hand column, the category called Usually Bladder Friendly—unless there's a food on that list you know to be irritating to you, which you obviously should avoid. But eat only from that category, nothing at all from Foods Worth Trying or Foods to Avoid. And when we say *only*, we mean without exception, without a single lapse for the entire eight weeks. In addition, for those eight weeks, avoid multivitamins, which have the common irritants of vitamin B and potassium, bottled drinks with added electrolytes, all over-the-counter medications (unless prescribed by a doctor), and any supplement you tend to buy from a health food store or acupuncturist. Multivitamins and the waters you buy at the gym invariably contain potassium. Over-the-counter medications, unless prescribed by a doctor, typically contain acidic or potassium-rich binders. And such "health" supplements as turmeric, for example, which you might be adding to your diet as an anti-inflammatory, can be acidic and thus irritating to the bladder. Remember too that carbonated beverages, no matter how healthy they "look," are irritants: The bubbles are acidic and irritate the bladder. Basically, in these eight weeks of "pure" eating, you will create a clean template on which you can create a new model of eating that will let you heal.

After this eight-week period, it will be time to start testing foods you have been assiduously avoiding and possibly missing from the Foods Worth Trying and Foods to Avoid columns to see if they will work in your diet in the future. This testing can be an elaborate process, and it does take time, primarily because you must do it *one food at a time, one test per week*. Reintroduce each one into your diet for three or four days in a row and see what happens, then stop using it, then wait till the following week before trying the next Food Worth Trying or Food to Avoid item. Can't figure out how you lived without coffee for the past month and a half? Ease into it with the low-acid version from the Worth Trying column—and just for three or four days. Then discontinue the coffee, and wait a few days before you reintroduce another food to test how it goes.

"How it goes" means asking whether, after the three or four days of a reintroduced food, you sense any difference in urinary symptoms. Any bloat? Abdominal pain? Intestinal discomfort? Vaginal symptoms? Record the change. Again, wait a few days, introduce another favorite from the list for another three or four days, then stop for two to three days and record any changes.

Do the same week after week. Do it conscientiously. "Sort of" following this regimen does not work. Neither does trying to replace the avoidance diet with your physical therapy regimen. As we noted earlier, dietary change and PT are not an either/or approach to the chronic pelvic discomfort of painful bladder syndrome. The PT techniques you'll read about below don't take the place of avoiding foods that aggravate your bladder—and vice versa. You need both.

So yes, the "research" you do on what irritates and what does not irritate takes a lot of time, but your body took a lot of time to get where it is, and it won't get better in just a few weeks, or even in a few months. The point is to take the time that's needed to adjust your diet so that you can eat without it resulting in discomfort or pain.

Iris has found that approximately half of her patients recognize symptom changes and adjust their eating to capture improvements in the way they feel after about six weeks of the eight, if they have been assiduous. And she is pretty sure that for those who don't see any alteration in the way foods affect their symptoms, it is because their bodies are still so upregulated by so many other drivers of pain that they simply are unable to recognize change as it happens. Avoidance of the foods that irritate your bladder *will* work in time.

The Most Bothersome Foods for PBS Patients with Endo:

Carbonated beverages—including clear sparkling waters

Sodas, diet or regular, caffeinated or caffeine-free

Tomatoes

Citrus fruits

Coffee, decaf or regular

Alcohol

Chocolate

Green tea

Spicy food

B-complex vitamins

Cranberry juice

Electrolyte waters

PHYSICAL THERAPY

The good news about doing PT for pelvic pain associated with PBS is that the response from the bladder comes pretty fast for many of the symptoms. The irritation will cool down fairly quickly, the relief will be noticeable, and the discomfort will continually diminish as you continue the therapy.

The treatment we recommend includes specific manual therapy techniques and neuromuscular reeducation under the care of a qualified physical therapist, plus exercises you can do on your own—namely, the Basic Six from chapter 3, which you should be doing every day as a matter of course, as well as some simple techniques for retraining the bladder.

Working with a Professional

Manual techniques for PBS will center around the bladder, urethra, abdomen, thighs, and pelvic floor. Myofascial trigger point release and visceral mobilization or manipulation, both internal and external, can release the restricted tissue and subsequently the surrounding organs.

In addition, a few muscle groups—specifically, the urethral sphincters that control the release of urine, the obturator internus on the sidewall of the pelvic floor that can pull on the urethra or bladder (or can become a trigger point or cause nerve irritation), and the levator ani, connected to the tailbone—can, if tightened, increase bladder frequency, urgency, incomplete emptying, and pain. Restrictions in all of these muscles can be loosened through manipulation and mobilization to ease the bladder frequency, urgency, and pain. By the way, the obturator internus is also a hip rotator, which is why hip problems sometimes can cause bladder issues.

Also, even where endo is the primary cause of the bladder dysfunction, abdominal muscles may also be affected thanks to viscero-somatic cross-talk, which then affects the bladder itself via somato-visceral cross-talk. Muscle manipulation or mobilization will also ease the restrictions in this muscle group.

On Your Own

For painful bladder syndrome, we offer an edit to the frequency and suggested number of repetitions of the Basic Six exercises. In addition—and most important—every time you feel any symptom at all, do any two of these exercises right then, in the moment. You should of course continue to do all of the Basic Six every day; be sure to accompany Exercises 2 through 6 with the deep breathing of Exercise 1.

Exercise 1: Breathe—5 reps 5 times a day

Exercise 2: Pelvic Floor Drop—2 reps every hour

Exercise 3: Pelvic Floor Stretch—2 or 3 reps twice a day

Exercise 4: Hip Rotator Stretch—2 or 3 reps twice a day

Exercise 5: Hip Flexor Stretch—2 to 4 reps a day

Exercise 6: Abdominal Stretch—2 to 4 reps a day

In addition, the following seven bladder retraining techniques can make a substantive difference in relieving pain and discomfort and in undoing the lifestyle limitations imposed by urinary frequency/urgency and the other effects of painful bladder syndrome. You probably want to practice them at home till you feel comfortable enough to rely on them "in public":

1. The moment you feel the first inkling of the urge to urinate, do the Pelvic Floor Drop, Exercise 2 of the Basic Six. Start

with that deep inhalation that expands the abdomen and the ribs as you let your pelvic floor "open" and relax the muscles in your lower abdomen around the bladder. Obviously, precisely because urgency may be an issue you are confronting, you could find yourself doing this retraining exercise many, many times a day. That is good. Practice makes perfect, and while patience will be required, you should see a difference within three to four weeks. A mentor of Amy's used to set an alarm—with a beeper—at ten-minute intervals, as a reminder to practice this exercise. It was totally annoying until the mentor realized how well it worked—well enough to extend the timing of the intervals and, in due course, to not need either the alarm or the exercise reminder at all. The best retraining tool is clearly the one that becomes unnecessary because the bladder has been retrained! So once you do see a difference, that is your cue to keep it up; at the first sensation of the need to urinate, default to Exercise 2 of the Basic Six.

2. As an "and/or" to that first retraining tip, the moment you feel the urge to urinate, do the Pelvic Floor Stretch, Exercise 3 of the Basic Six—if you can. If you're at work or somewhere else where doing that exercise is not possible or convenient, do Exercise 5, the Hip Flexor Stretch.

3. Distract yourself mentally. Really. Think of something relaxing: Send your mind to your favorite place in the world, with your favorite person. Go mentally to whatever place or situation makes you feel calm. Concentrate on that till you feel your body relaxing too.

4. Practice mimicking the muscle release that precedes urination. Close your eyes, imagine the moment of relief you feel just as the flow begins. Let it happen.

5. After urinating but while still on the toilet, do repeated Pelvic Floor Drops with deep breathing for six to eight breaths. This allows the bladder to relax and to empty fully.

6. Don't strain or push the urine out. Instead, relax and breathe.

7. If these six techniques don't work for you, try doing several quick pelvic floor contractions, let go, and be sure to breathe deeply. The downside is that over time, this may tighten the muscles further, so use this technique sparingly and only if all else fails.

5

ENDO AND
THE GI TRACT

The gastrointestinal tract—your gut—functions as the center of your body's digestive system. It occupies the same geography as the bladder—namely, the abdomino-pelvic cavity. Like the bladder, the GI organs are secured between the diaphragm and the pelvis and are enclosed by the spinal column and by all the surrounding muscles that protect the organs and that you need for urinating, defecating, giving birth, throwing up, singing, and coughing.* Although technically the GI tract extends from the mouth to the anus, the main organs of digestion—namely, the colon or large intestine, the small intestine or small bowel, and the rectum—sit together, functioning in continuity, in that crowded cavity.

By now, you have an idea of what endometriosis can do to

* The abdomino-pelvic cavity also contains your liver, pancreas, spleen, kidneys, and adrenal glands.

these organs. Unlike the cells of the uterine lining, which flow out of the body during menstruation, endo cells do not dissipate through a natural exit; rather, they thicken and expand. As they do, these implants affect both the organs they are growing on or adjacent to and the muscles and fascia that underlie the organs. Their presence on the organ wall or adjacent to the organ makes the organs adhere to one another, while their pulling on the underlying muscles and fascia tenses and tightens them disproportionately to one side. The anatomical distortion and the inflammation trigger dysfunction and its accompanying symptoms.

Endo implants on or near the GI tract can cause diarrhea, constipation, bloating, painful bowel movements, and abdominal pain, all of which are sufficiently uncomfortable and unpredictable as to be life-limiting. The resultant pulling and tugging on the fascia and muscles can prevent the bowel's normal peristalsis and can slow its motility, causing constipation that may be painful and is equally life-limiting. When the constipation is so "obstinate" as to be virtually intractable, enabling only rare release of watery stool, GI specialists refer to it as obstipation.

Meanwhile, the inflammation of endo plus the slowdown of bowel motility mean that the bacteria of the small intestine stay there for a long time, during which they fester and grow well beyond what is normal. That condition is called small intestinal bacterial overgrowth (SIBO), and it can impede the absorption of nutrients into the bloodstream and release enzymes and gases that cause bloat and pain as well as diarrhea. To the triplets identified in the previous chapter—endo, painful bladder syndrome, and musculoskeletal dysfunction—we now add a quadruplet—namely, SIBO.

Gastrointestinal Pain and Discomfort, in Patients' Words:

"So bloated I look like I'm five months pregnant..."

"Alternating constipation and diarrhea..."

"It feels like reflux..."

"A feeling of fullness in the rectum..."

"I'm so nauseous I feel like I want to vomit..."

"I need to put my feet up on the toilet seat to get my bowels moving..."

"A burning pain..."

"I have to move around on the toilet to get a bowel movement going..."

"I sometimes need to use my finger to start a bowel movement..."

"A sharp pain with bowel movements..."

"I never feel really empty..."

"It takes me nearly half an hour on the toilet before I can move my bowels..."

In some women, these symptoms occur at random. In others, they occur in sync with a woman's cycle; after being constipated for two or three weeks, the arrival of the menstrual flow metaphorically pops a cork in these women, and liquid stool just pours out of them. And then the cycle begins again. But even if these events occur only sporadically, the fact of their recurrence is a signal that endo could well be the cause.

Dr. Laurence Orbuch, Iris's husband and a gynecologist who

specializes in endometriosis, says that for his endo patients, the most common non-gynecological symptoms they present with are GI symptoms. In one key study, a full 90 percent of women with endo presented with GI symptoms—and, it is important to note, only 7.6 percent of the women had implants on the bowel itself.[11] Dr. Orbuch, well known for grand rounds presentations that educate hospital GI staff about endo, suggests that the diagnosis of GI disorders, especially SIBO, should be considered a "red flag" by healthcare providers, signaling the possibility—if not the likelihood—of endometriosis as an underlying cause.

But as with women presenting with urological symptoms, this connection is all too often missed. In fact, in what might be considered a paradigm for both the ongoing silos within medicine *and* for that twelve-year gap between first symptoms and a diagnosis of endo, women with these GI symptoms typically first see their internist, are then referred to a gastroenterologist who performs endoscopy that is typically normal, after which they are diagnosed with irritable bowel syndrome (IBS) and are prescribed medications that decrease their bloating or increase their bowel motility. The relief tends to be temporary, but the underlying cause has actually gone unrecognized, leaving the poor patient blind to what is fundamentally wrong. The problem, says Dr. Orbuch, is that the view through the specialist's lens too often results only in treating symptoms, not in ascertaining their cause.

Dr. Leo Treyzon is the rare gastroenterology specialist who *does* seek to find the cause behind patients' symptoms. He is the exemplar of a GI doc who knows that the GI tract that is his specialty does not operate in isolation and therefore requires a whole-body approach. It means that Treyzon doesn't rely on endoscopy alone to tell him what may be going on in a patient's GI tract. It also means that he understands the connection between GI tract dysfunction and endometriosis and is acutely aware of their potential coexistence in his female patients. Treyzon is meticulous and insistent in asking patients to chronicle and catalogue their pain. He listens carefully and reads the meaning in what patients tell him.

Very few gastroenterologists query their patients about *muscle* pain; Treyzon makes a point of doing so. "People who are constipated typically have to push and strain in order to evacuate," he says, "and because endo is chronic, the pushing and straining can overwork the muscles," tightening the pelvic and abdominal muscles significantly. That muscle pain is a clue that endo may be present.

There are others. For example, says Treyzon, nerve fibers in the bowel, if invaded by endo, can cause the patient to feel "something" irritating in the colon or small bowel. Equally, if there is endo around the rectum, the patient may feel a phantom sensation of needing to evacuate, which then proves futile.

Pain sensitization, which becomes progressively more widespread and more irritating, is a key issue Treyzon typically explores—even though, like muscle pain, the central nervous system is not conventionally thought of as a gastroenterology concern. "If a patient is always in discomfort," he explains, "the nerves become hyperaware, and the pain pathways are altered." Where there is endo, this can create situations where the pain feels "outsized"—for example, bloating or gas far worse than normal, as experienced by the patient claiming that her gut was so distended she was sure she looked five months pregnant. That augmentation of pain awareness is a signal of endo, Treyzon says.

We've seen this before. By now, it's an old and familiar story: muscle pain in the abdomen, bladder pain and discomfort, and now widening problems with digestion and gastrointestinal dysfunction. In each case, well-trained and well-meaning specialists in their separate disciplines rarely if ever consider that endometriosis might be a cause; they miss the bigger picture of how a patient's symptoms might be connected to a disease that lies outside of their discipline. Where GI issues are concerned, they instead tend to plot a course of treatment for IBS, which, patients are told, cannot be discerned through any known test or imaging, is incurable, and is chronic. Dr. Orbuch and Dr. Treyzon are the rare exceptions who have come out of their silos to treat not separate physiological systems, but humans with totally interconnected physiological systems.

But for most women, the general rule, not exceptions like Orbuch and Treyzon, prevails, and the results are typically unhappy at best. Presenting with a prevalence of GI symptoms, albeit with no underlying GI cause, and "labeled" in her twenties or thirties as someone with IBS, a woman will eventually learn to live with the symptoms, to "work around" them, to "normalize" the experience. But the truth is that IBS is a catchall diagnosis, and the medical profession's failure to dig further into the etiology of such symptoms, especially in young women, is an evasion that can leave the patient feeling powerless against "the luck of the draw."

The practical implications of this, for both doctors and patients, are profound. A colleague of Iris's since her fellowship and a co-author with her on a key paper[12] is yet another doctor named Orbuch—gastroenterologist Dr. Murray Orbuch, brother to Laurence, brother-in-law to Iris. Deep medical curiosity buttressed by extensive training at the National Institutes of Health forms a commitment, shared with his brother, to dig deep into the etiology of women's symptoms. Murray Orbuch puts the case well—namely, until it is universally recognized that "what is sometimes taken as IBS is not just IBS, it behooves both the gynecologist and the gastroenterologist to ask about painful periods, pain during sex, pain during bowel movements." And where any such gynecological symptoms are part of the overall constellation, they should instantly trigger further investigation.

For women—especially young women, since "IBS presents early in life"—an IBS diagnosis should therefore reverberate as an important signal that other, deeper causes may also be at issue. To borrow gastroenterologist Orbuch's acutely apt verb, it *behooves* "any young woman with painful periods" who has received a diagnosis of IBS to insist on further investigation. Patients have an obligation to question a diagnosis and to educate themselves about what doctors tell them; it is why we have written this book.* You have only one body and one life—and you deserve to find out what is really going on.

THE MUSCULOSKELETAL CONNECTION

Just as with bladder issues, when GI issues are present, the impact on the musculoskeletal system can be painful and distressing. Endo implants growing near or on the organs within the crowded cavity irritate and restrict the muscles that "govern" bowel function, and muscles that have become restricted "reply" back through somato-visceral cross-talk and further affect dysfunction in the organs and cause more pain.

These muscles, the muscles that control and enable bowel function, include the internal and external anal sphincters and the pelvic floor muscles. The internal anal sphincter is an *involuntary* muscle in the anus that holds feces within the rectum; obviously, it stays contracted most of the time, but when the rectum is full, the fullness triggers nerves that cause the anus to relax and open. The external anal sphincter is a *voluntary* muscle that you willfully

---

* For internet sites you can trust, consult our Resources section (page 259).

contract in order to hold the feces inside you until you get to a toilet. The pelvic floor muscles, which comprise the sling around the end of the rectum, are also voluntary muscles; you control them to govern when you will allow the feces to descend from the rectum toward the anus and thereby out of your body. Actually, the puborectalis muscle, a muscle that is situated at an angle to the rectum, is what relaxes to allow the feces to descend. (When we are upright, this muscle kinks the rectum, closing it off so that stool does not leak out; we remain continent.) If the pelvic floor muscles get tightened by endo implants, as they frequently do, the puborectalis can't relax, the angle stays acute, the muscle won't open, and you will feel constipated and probably bloated.

In fact, with the entire abdomino-pelvic cavity virtually filled by the GI tract, viscero-somatic reflexes from anywhere in the cavity can affect musculoskeletal real estate ranging from the ribs down to the pelvic floor. And all of those tensed, restricted muscles, in their turn, can send it right back to the colon and bowel and rectum.

BEATING ENDO THAT AFFECTS THE GI TRACT: THE BASIC TOOLS

As always with endo, the methodology is to deal with each of the conditions you experience as symptoms, and certainly, prescription medications are among the tools that can relieve or at least mitigate a number of GI symptoms. SIBO, for example, can be successfully treated with oral antibiotics that stay within the small bowel. These are not the kinds of antibiotics that will wreak havoc with your gut. For example, they are nothing like the antibiotics people routinely take for sinus infections, strep throat, and so forth. Yes, there are some people who cannot tolerate the antibiotics for SIBO, but most can, and this is therefore a safe and effective treatment that will remove one of the symptoms and thereby eliminate one instigator, at least, of nervous system sensitization. Iris cautions that most endo patients will require two or even three rounds of antibiotics to treat SIBO because their inflammation has been present for such a long time. Excision surgery, once the body has cooled, will remove the inflammation that ignites the SIBO.

Moreover, since digestion is the function at issue, what you eat can also affect many aspects of the discomfort you experience. Overall, beating endo will call for an anti-inflammatory nutrition plan, as we will detail further in chapter 8, but there are also certain foods to avoid and others to embrace to calm down a troubled GI tract. Obviously, the list of foods that will help a condition characterized by constipation will be very different from the list of foods that will help a condition of diarrhea. If constipation is your problem, you want to eat more fiber, but make it organic, soluble fiber foods like the inside of fruits—avoid the skin—and cooked vegetables, only adding such insoluble, gas-producing fiber foods as beans and legumes, oat bran, and cruciferous vegetables once your gut has begun to calm down. And any time you increase your intake of fiber, it is important to increase your intake of water as well.

If diarrhea is the issue, you can take a supplement that bulks the stool—psyllium husk, for example—and drink plenty of water. Milk products, fried or greasy foods, caffeine, alcohol, acidic foods, even eggs and chocolate can irritate the bowel. Some foods can thicken the stool and slow bowel motility; others loosen the stool and may stimulate the bowels. Your physician or a range of internet sites can supply you with lists of these categories of food.

There are some simple ways to help alleviate the pain and discomfort far too many women experience in conjunction with bowel movements. One old standby of pain relief is a simple heating pad placed on the abdomen. Another is to adjust your bowel habits to those of our foremothers—and to much of the contemporary non-Western world—and assume a squatting position when you defecate. A toilet stool can be useful for this, the best-known commercial variant being the Squatty Potty. But however you approach it, the squatting position beats sitting as a way to ease the process and ensure that it is completed efficiently and effectively. The reason is simple: Sitting on a toilet kinks the aforementioned puborectalis muscle, puts pressure on the rectum, effectively plugs the pathway out of the rectum, and forces you to strain. Squatting keeps the puborectalis muscle in line and enables complete elimination. Whatever method you choose, the aim is for your knees to be elevated above your hips.

If circumstances don't let you manage a squatting position, at least try to avoid straining. Instead, tighten your *abdominal* muscles. There's a process we call hardbelly-softbelly. Basically, while seated on the toilet, take a deep breath, and as you exhale, tighten your abdominal wall and then instantly mimic what happens when you release your urine; this opens the sphincters. Repeat this alternating hardbelly-softbelly movement until you successfully empty your bowels. If you still have trouble, you might try a method that Amy teaches, which her patients have dubbed the I Love You massage (see box at right). This technique for an easier elimination with less pain takes its name from the letters *ILU*—the letters whose shapes you will trace as you do the massage. Minimal as it seems, the ILU massage can have a profound impact on a sluggish colon, and even if you have no discomfort at all, it is a fine way to relax your body's core. The relaxation that can result is an additional tool for bringing the central nervous system out of fight-or-flight mode, which slows the colon down, and into rest-and-digest mode, which tells the colon to get a move on.

The I Love You Massage

How to do it:

Flatten your palm, make a fist, or use your fingers, first to trace the letter *I* in a descending movement from just under your left rib cage to your pelvic bone. Do this ten to fifteen times. Then place your palm, fist, or fingers under the right rib cage and draw the *L*— right to left horizontally, then straight down to the pubic bone. Again, do this ten to fifteen times. Finally, the *U*: Start on the right, at the top edge of the pelvic bone, and massage up toward the rib cage, then left across the body, then down to the top of the pelvic bone. Do this ten to fifteen times as well. What you have done is massage the descending colon, the transverse colon, and the ascending colon, thus stimulating the involuntary contractions that actually move the stool. Use moderate pressure; if it hurts, lighten the pressure. If it still hurts, stop—although even a light massage may cause some soreness at first.

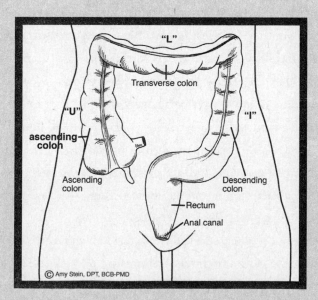

Another key technique for achieving complete emptying and for addressing your pain and bloating is, very simply, helping the emptying along. You can do this in the shower or while lying in bed on either side. Apply a small amount of lubricant—any kind at all—to your chosen finger, practice some deep breathing, find the anal opening, and then gently and slowly insert the lubricated finger into your rectum. Press the finger in four different directions—north, south, east, west (or, if you prefer: noon, three o'clock, six o'clock, nine o'clock), holding each direction for ten deep breaths as you gradually increase the pressure. This action relaxes certain pelvic floor muscles and thus alerts the colon to move stool down to the rectum, from which it can now be easily eliminated. Retract your finger. Caution: If you feel any pain or discomfort, ease the pressure, and if the pain or discomfort continues, stop entirely—and then consult with your physical therapist.

Moreover, virtually all of the exercises offered on pages 69 to 74 will help lessen the tightness, pain, and bloating of bowel dysfunction as well. At the same time, it is also essential to maintain physical activity. Whether you walk, or run, or participate in a sport or recreation you love, increasing your heart rate on a sustained basis is as essential for GI health as it is for bladder health and, indeed, for overall health. Start small, then do more, then do even more, then continue to move your body every day.

In addition to what you can do yourself, pelvic floor PT specialists can release the trigger points in all these muscles of the abdomino-pelvic cavity, and muscles thus released can "talk back" to the organs affected by endo, "telling" them to relax so they can do the jobs they were designed to do.

These and other nonsurgical treatments have the effect of downregulating the central nervous system too, and an endo specialist like Iris will continually monitor the improvements of symptoms that these treatments effect, isolating out each underlying cause until only the endo is left. Only then can she begin to ready the patient for the surgery, if needed, that will excise the implants.

As always, it's essential to keep in mind that the dysfunction did not begin in a vacuum, and that it will take time to reverse a GI tract that has been dysfunctional for years. SIBO, musculoskeletal issues, and distortions to the anatomy from endo implants are not isolated instances that can be defined in separate diagnoses and addressed with individual treatments. Where GI symptoms are concerned, they are but one part of a larger story, and the healthcare practitioner assessing your GI symptoms needs to take them all into consideration.

ENDO AND SEX

Can endometriosis affect a woman's sex life? You bet it can—and it does so all too frequently.

The simple and unhappy fact is that sexual dysfunction and the pain it causes are common symptoms of the endo disease process and afflict most endo sufferers. The dysfunction derives from the distortion of the pelvic anatomy caused by thickening endo implants and the scarring and adhesions the implants produce—all exacerbated by the viscero-somatic cross-talk from any of the organs in the pelvis to surrounding muscles and tissue. In addition, the muscle clenching that happens reflexively "against" the distortion and the scarring can affect the ability of muscles to respond, and compromised ligaments can restrict movement within the abdomino-pelvic cavity. This in turn can affect the endo sufferer's responsiveness.

But it is important to note that what hurts first and foremost is penetration itself—the penis pushing on the endo implants. The pain can be particularly severe in the area behind the cervix, the precise area where penetration is deepest. In time, as the entire pelvic floor tightens up against the anatomical distortions—and as constipation typically exacerbates the situation—entry itself becomes so painful that penetration becomes almost literally impossible. Unhappily, hormonal changes induced by a number of endo treatments can actually amplify the pain.

The impact on a woman's life—and on her relationship with a partner—can be profound. Experiencing sex that hurts is likely to raise a woman's stress quotient and/or lead to reluctance to engage, which affects a partner as well. Over time, reluctance can lead to avoidance, further straining the relationship and taking a serious toll on both partners—which is not good for anyone's health.

The dysfunction may not be confined to the act of sexual intercourse alone; pain can make it difficult for a woman to use a tampon during her period or, with fairly profound ramifications, may cause her to avoid undergoing a gynecological examination.

Understanding all this and knowing precisely how endo can affect sexual activity are essential to addressing the issue and restoring sexual health.

THE PAIN

The medical term for pain with penetrative sex is *dyspareunia*; pain with or without touch at the opening to the vagina is called *vestibulodynia*.

The vestibule is where the vulva, the external part of your genitalia, meets or actually surrounds the vaginal opening. It's a protective and therefore highly sensitive part of the female anatomy, filled with nerve fibers and susceptible to a range of highly individual pain responses. In some women with endometriosis, vestibulodynia may actually be present all the time, affecting them so severely that they cannot wear tight clothing or sit at all, much less experience touch or penetration.

Dyspareunia may be superficial, affecting primarily the external tissues and muscles of the vagina, or deep, if penetration applies pressure to implants behind the cervix and in the uterosacral ligaments, both of which are typical and frequent sites of such implants.

It's not hard to imagine endo's impact on the anatomy of the abdomino-pelvic area and how it can make everything inside the area stop moving and working the way it should. Now think specifically about the effect of endo implants near or on the sex organs. Imagine those implants pulling on the surrounding tissue and restricting that tissue from sliding and gliding as tissue should. When the tissues of the organs of sexual function are just not moving, sex is going to hurt. And when the penis—or a finger or a wand or toy or any object—pushes on the cul-de-sac infiltrated with endometriosis, sex definitely hurts.

In response to the pain, your body will tend to clench, actually promoting further pain, while the number of nerves also multiplies. This of course magnifies the sensitivity to touch even further. It's another instance of intense response to pain causing even worse pain. The nerves irritated by the endo typically innervate other nerves stretching from the vulva to the deepest part of the pelvic floor, thereby passing the message of pain throughout the muscles and tissue along the route of sexual penetration.

The pudendal nerve, the main nerve of the body's erogenous zone, typically transmits much of this pain. This nerve innervates most of the pelvic floor muscles and thus also affects bladder, bowel, and sexual functions. Actually a pair of nerves at the midpoint of the pelvis, one on either side of the body, the pudendal nerve carries sensation and supplies motor energy along a winding path starting in the sacrum, passing out the back of the pelvis through muscles and ligaments, sweeping around and then swerving through the pelvis, and ending in the region of the clitoris, vulva, and anus. If any portion of it becomes irritated, it can wreak havoc throughout the pelvic floor and in the genitals. Its variety of pain sensations—burning heat, itching, cold, shooting pain, razor-like sharpness—may range throughout the abdomen and into the groin and buttocks as well as down the legs, making it sometimes painful to sit down while also exacerbating bladder and GI dysfunctions. All this in addition to rendering sex painful.

Painful Sex, in Patients' Words:

"At first, it feels okay, but if it goes any deeper, it's like I'm being hit…"

"A raw, burning feeling…"

"It hurts during and sometimes for hours after sex—even for days…"

"It's like my partner hits a wall…"

"Feels like a razor slicing me…"

"I'm debilitated for days afterward…"

"I can't have sex. Period…"

"I feel like I'm tearing, even though my gyno said the tissues look fine…"

Little wonder that for many women thus affected by endo, penetrative sex, arguably one of life's most fundamental pleasures and a pretty essential glue of couplehood, simply becomes too painful altogether. Postponing or evading or totally copping out of sex because of worry over the anticipated pain can become sheer fear over the mere thought of sex; this can actually bring on the pain itself, while it also creates a level of anxiety that becomes its own health condition. It is what psychologists call "fear avoidance," and it can get so built into the psyche that it turns into a separate source of chronic musculoskeletal pain—persistent and hard to undo.

Ironically and sadly, it isn't just the presence of endo implants that can engender this distress in the pelvic area; many of the medications used to treat endo are also complicit. Birth control pills, for example, regularly prescribed as a "pain medication" for the severe menstrual cramps of endo, as well as a number of the hormonal creams often prescribed for daily use, act by "shutting off the ovaries so that they stop making estrogen and dramatically decrease the amount of testosterone produced," in the words of Dr. Andrew T. Goldstein, a specialist in women's sexual health as practitioner, researcher, and teacher.[13] In fact, Goldstein continues, birth control pills produce a "75 percent reduction in free testosterone," defined as the amount of testosterone that's available to the cells—which is precisely what the pills are intended to do.

For women with endo, one result is a lessening of the pain, but there are other consequences as well. What Goldstein calculates as "a relatively large minority" of women on birth control pills may confront sexual dysfunctions ranging from a lowering of desire to deficient lubrication to decreased orgasm to pain during sex. Especially at the vaginal opening in the vulvar vestibule, the tissue, says Goldstein, "is very testosterone-dependent," so the drop in testosterone caused by the medication can affect the integrity of that tissue. That's why some doctors recommend testosterone cream to counter the dryness of the tissue, as dryness can make penetration by a partner both difficult and painful. Lupron, a well-known but infamous endo medication, likewise suppresses the body's production of estrogen and can thus parch the tissue of the genitals, setting the stage for painful intercourse. The instinctive response to the pain—the reflexive clenching and tightening of the pelvic muscles—can render penetration yet more difficult.

For the woman suffering from endo but finding some mitigation of her suffering through medication, this makes for bitter assessments and some trade-offs. Will you give up sex in order to be free of chronic pelvic pain? Which pleasure are you willing to trade away: freedom from chronic pelvic pain or intimacy with a partner? How much pain are you willing to put up with for what kind of pleasure? We've written this book to keep you from ever having to face such dilemmas, for whichever choice you make constitutes a narrowing of life.

What's a woman to do? You are likely in your late teens, twenties or thirties or forties, at a time of life that you've been told is your "sexual prime," and thanks to a bunch of endo implants growing somewhere inside you and the medication you are taking to assuage their damage, it has become painful to have sex. Our goal for our readers as for our patients is penetrative sex—joyful penetrative sex—and we want to share with you some of the best ways we know of to accomplish that goal. But it cannot be regained overnight, so take advantage of a goodly number of options along the way until PT and the right surgery achieve the results both you and we want. Of course, talk to your doctor or maybe a sex therapist or go online. There are many possibilities. After all, trouble with sex is not a new issue; people have been writing advice books on the subject for thousands of years. But along with the many options, some caveats are in order as well.

LUBRICANTS

Apart from the medicinal vaginal creams some women apply daily, there are the standard creams and oils to "replenish" vaginal moisture, as the ads often claim. It is a simple and basic notion: The oil or cream serves as a lubricant to ease penetration. The potential downside of these lubricants is that many of them may contain ingredients that affect the treatment you are undergoing for endometriosis or that directly impact the vulvar tissue—in which case you can find yourself helping one life-limiting condition while simultaneously initiating another.

In fact, it is essential to check the ingredients your chosen lubricant contains for all sorts of reasons. Some ingredients can irritate the tissue in various ways. For example, the vaginal canal has a certain pH balance, which is the measure of its acidity or alkalinity, and it is a measure that should be maintained for optimal health. In fact, a pH imbalance raises susceptibility to yeast infections. Propylene glycol, a common ingredient in a number of lubricants—for example, K-Y Jelly—is something we both consider a no-no; it may throw off the pH balance and can potentially irritate the vaginal tissue. You'll be interested to know that its primary industrial use is as a de-icing agent. In addition to propylene glycol, parabens are occasionally found in lubricants, but as they are carcinogenic, you want to avoid those products as much as possible.

Fortunately, these days a variety of better choices is available. You can now find propylene glycol–free, paraben-free, pH-balanced lubricants, all advertising the ingredients they do *not* contain. (Check our recommendations in the Resources section; page 259.) We also recommend going back to basics and simply using coconut oil or olive oil as lubricants—the latter because it is a good lubricant and something you probably have in your kitchen, the former because it contains anti-inflammatory compounds that won't compromise the medication you are taking. Keep in mind, however, that both these oils are likely to break down latex, so if condoms are your go-to method of birth control, you will likely need to find a replacement.

POSITION

Yes, position *does* count. Simply put, some positions for having sex tend to cause less pain than others. Two soaringly credentialed physical therapists, Hollis Herman and Kathe Wallace, founders of the Herman & Wallace Pelvic Rehabilitation Institute, recommend a number of positions as "good" for painful intercourse, and here are six samples that a number of Amy's patients in particular have found useful. But since this is a highly individual matter, it is important to note that one, some, all, or none of these may work for you.[14]

Recommended Positions for Women Who Suffer from Pain during Penetrative Sex

POSITION 1: The woman lies on her back with knees bent up, her hips apart and supported by pillows on the outside of the knees; the partner is between her legs, supported on hands.

POSITION 2: The woman lies on her back with hips in a neutral position, possibly with her back supported by a towel; the partner straddles the woman and is supported on elbows or hands.

POSITION 3: The partner lies on his or her back, with legs inside the woman's. She straddles her partner facing forward, her hips and knees bent upward and her back neutral, flexed, or extended. In this position, pillows on her partner's thighs can be used to control the depth of penetration.

POSITION 4: The woman lies on her stomach with or without a pillow under her lower belly. Her partner straddles her, with the woman's legs inside her partner's, enabling vaginal entry from the rear. This position should *not* be used if you experience deep cervix pain.

POSITION 5: The woman sits on a chair or sofa facing forward, with hips apart and back neutral. Her partner is on top with legs inside the woman's for frontal entry.

POSITION 6: The partner lies on his or her back with legs inside the woman's. She is on top, facing backward and straddling the partner, enabling vaginal entry from the rear.

In addition, there are products now available that help with deep penetrative pain, allowing the partner to enter only at a certain depth. One brand that Amy likes and recommends is the Ohnut company. Check it out in our Resources section (page 259).

PHYSICAL THERAPY

The one thing that is commonly able to address painful sex effectively is physical therapy. It cannot, of course, affect the hormonal tinkering that medications typically cause. Expecting PT to solve that issue is "like changing the tires to fix the carburetor," in Dr. Goldstein's words—i.e., these are two different problems. But PT can often diminish the dyspareunia in superficial tissues and muscles, can lessen the deeper musculoskeletal tightening and damage, and can abate the sensitivity to both touch and penetration.*

The specialized pelvic floor physical therapy that is so central to our multimodal approach is acutely well equipped to tackle the musculoskeletal effects that can make for painful sex. It can work whether those effects result from nerve irritation that may create pain or spasm as the patient guards against the irritation, or from any other cause. Obviously, the physical therapist first needs to identify the specific area being affected and to determine what is being restricted, what is in spasm, and which nerves are being irritated.

Once that analysis has been completed, the various techniques of pelvic floor PT come into play. For the pain, that would include the skilled techniques of a pelvic floor physical therapist, including mobilization of connective tissue around the pudendal and pelvic nerves as well as in surrounding muscles and fascia, myofascial trigger point release, and calming muscle reflexes. The PT would also include techniques to expand range of motion and to carefully strengthen the muscles of the core—which can in turn diminish the pain of sexual activity and, equally, the hesitation and thus the guarding against such activity.

Certain implements, usually assisted by lubricants, can supple-

---

* Be aware that as of this writing, medical insurance providers will not cover PT for sexual dysfunction *per se* but will cover PT to enable a woman to undergo a gynecological examination. Providers attribute the former dysfunction to "recreational" causes and do not consider it a health issue. Changing this false and misleading designation would save insurance providers a great deal of money—and their customers a great deal of pain and puzzlement.

ment the physical therapist's treatment of sexual dysfunction. If the pain of sex occurs at the vestibule because the tissue cannot be stretched without causing pain, a physical therapist might well suggest the use of a dilator to widen the opening, and if the issue is myofascial trigger points, superficial or deep, a therapeutic wand may be recommended. Physical therapists use both, very cautiously, when educating patients in the office about their home program; they show patients how to relax the muscles of the vestibule and to release superficial and deep trigger points. In widening the opening, the dilator is obviously aimed at easing penetration. The therapeutic wand can release a trigger point and can penetrate to reach a deep point of pain as the patient feels it. Dilators are typically purchased as a set in graduated widths and lengths. For women prone to yeast infections or urinary tract infections, the recommendation is to use dilators and wands made of glass, which is less susceptible to gathering bacteria, but if infection is not a worry, silicone implements are fine.

Amy and her team are highly circumspect in advising patients about the use of these implements and are diligent in demonstrating to patients in the office exactly how to use them at home. Patients are advised to use the implement on alternate days at first, especially if they are prone to irritation or are fearful, and they are required to return to the office and report on progress once a week. And for those women who are or who become comfortable using dilators and wands, Amy recommends keeping careful tabs on their use, continuing to revise their use, and to keep on advancing as your pain and hesitation diminish.

There is one more physical therapy technique we can recommend wholeheartedly for addressing painful sex, and that is deep breathing—both as a prelude to sexual activity and during the activity itself. We all know that the expectation or even the suspicion of imminent pain causes us to clench our muscles—including our pelvic floor muscles. Be aware of that as you contemplate having sex, and as preparation, try practicing the conscious breathing you learned in chapter 3. Start by inhaling slowly and from deep down for up to five seconds as you visualize the air expanding your belly outward and your ribs to the sides and as you let your pelvic floor "open." Then exhale for another five seconds or longer from the top down, letting the air flow out of your lungs and relaxing your ribs, belly, and pelvic floor. If you can, try to carry this breathwork into the sex as well. Breathe and open, breathe and open. Relax. Ease into it.

In relaxing tension and loosening muscles, physical therapy is an immensely powerful tool for making sex possible and pleasurable. And few things are more important than that to the goal of cooling the body and downregulating the central nervous system. But be aware that if deeply implanted endo is still pulling on the tissue and on the underlying muscles, organs, or fascia, and causing pain, those implants will need to be excised if the woman is to be restored to the full experience of penetrative sex—the essential goal. Iris says that it is the first thing her patients thank her for after surgery.

ALL KINDS OF INTIMACY

We also both advance the idea that there are many ways other than sexual intercourse to enjoy intimacy with your partner. We don't want you to settle. We want you to have a healthy sex life with, as noted, healthy penetrative sex. But as you go through the program this book presents, remember that there are multiple forms of intimacy.

As we all know, the most potent sex organ is the brain, and you should be aware that there are mental healthcare providers who specialize in sexual dysfunction and sexual health counseling who can help you address and overcome the fear avoidance that may accompany the dysfunction.

But the brain is also where creativity resides, so use it, let your imagination run wild, recall your early sexual experiences, which may not have included penetration at all, remember how exciting it was to explore and "sample," and keep in mind that *substantive* foreplay is essential for relaxation of the pelvic floor and for lubrication. So, until penetrative sex can again become routine, or until surgery removes the implants, or until physical therapy or modifying your position or using lubrication or deep breathing has done what they all can do to alleviate painful sex, we urge you to devise your own pathways to real physical pleasure.

PAIN, DISEASE, AND THE CENTRAL NERVOUS SYSTEM

A Multimodal Strategy for a Multidimensional Disease

Pain happens in the central nervous system, the CNS. It really doesn't happen anywhere else. Not at the point of injury or damage, not on the itch you scratch, not in the tooth that aches, not in the muscles that endo sufferers may have tightened through years of clenching.

Instead, it happens in the brain via the spinal cord, the two components of the CNS, located in two separate but continuous cavities—the cranial cavity and the spinal cavity—on the back side of the body. The system has two tasks: to sense how the body is functioning and to respond. It both monitors and controls the body's performance, both perceives it and adjusts it. It is in a sense a nonstop communication apparatus, receiving sensory signals and sending back motor instructions. It receives information that your brain identifies as drops of rain on your skin, then sends motor signals that prompt your leg muscles to run for cover or your arm muscles to open an umbrella.

These facts are the basis of our program for beating endo. Irrespective of all other treatments for your disease, these facts equip you to defy this disease and break its hold on your life through actions you yourself undertake. They put the umbrella in your hands and give you the wherewithal to open it and keep it open.

So let's start by taking a closer look at the pain process.

The sensation of pain arises from a stimulus—some type of damage to the tissue of the body. This could be a paper cut on your finger, for example, or our old standby, your hand touching a hot stove. Nerve endings called nociceptors detect the stimulus, sense it as a possible danger (*noci-* means "harm"), and sound the alarm. This alarm causes a response in the body's peripheral nervous system, the PNS, which exists to connect and relay information between the CNS and the organs, limbs, bones, muscles, and skin that constitute the rest of your body. The nociceptors that alert the PNS fire off a relay process, handing off the danger signal to nerves along the line that leads to the central nervous system. They take the signal right into the spinal cord, then travel one or two segments up and down the cord—the organs, if you remember high school biology, are innervated by the spinal segments—and eventually rise, via two ascending pathways, to the brain.

The brain is where the pain is realized. The arrival of the stimulus-turned-nociceptive-message activates several information processing systems in the brain. One system senses and assesses the potential danger; another determines the nature, location, and intensity of the stimulus; a third is in charge of your emotional and behavioral response, even deciding whether the danger is relevant given the context. (If it determines the danger is not relevant, it will filter it out of your consciousness till it really counts.) That perceiving and interpreting of the message determine where and when you undergo the actual sensory experience—of aching or twingeing, discomfort or distress, soreness or agony, or of some level of hurt or suffering along a richly varied spectrum of sensations.

Then, via two descending pathways, motor neurons are dispatched from the brain down the spinal cord to that part of the body that will respond to the pain, mobilizing it to expend energy to execute the response. In the case of the paper cut, motor neurons incite you to say "Ouch!" and probably impel you to lick your finger; in the matter of the hot stove, they prompt you to mutter a curse and abruptly pull your hand off the stove; and in response to whatever is making you feel discomfort in your abdomen or pelvis, they induce you to curl into the fetal position and subconsciously guard against the pain by tightening your abdominal muscles, tensing your lower back and even your shoulder and neck muscles, and of course clenching your pelvic floor muscles.

That is how pain happens, wherever you feel it, however long it lasts. Certainly, pain comes in different strengths and sizes, exhibits different levels of intensity, shows up in different forms. It may be severe enough to send you to bed or mild enough to barely slow you down. It might be acute—a sudden but brief zap, like the paper cut or the hot stove—or chronic, lasting well beyond the moment of injury until it becomes a part of life.

Melissa Farmer, PhD,* a clinical psychologist and researcher

---

* Member of the International Association for the Study of Pain, scientific program committee chair for the International Society for the Study of Women's Sexual Health, and a member of the distinguished International Academy of Sex Research.

based at Northwestern University who focuses on how the brain "learns," points out that pain also may be different in its properties—its quality or character—depending on which part of the body gets innervated by the nociceptors carrying the signal about harm. Somatic nociceptors, which are part of the peripheral nervous system, innervate skin, muscle, and bone; the perception of pain that results from their firing may be characterized as closely linked to the original stimulus. In other words, this is pain that is perceived as beginning and ending in a distinctive way, and as possessing a clear and particular quality that can be plainly described—sharp or dull, burning or cold, a shooting pain or a mild pain. These are pretty specific nociceptors, so you feel the pain pretty close to that place on your skin or the muscle or bone where the tissue damage first happened, you feel it start and finish up, and you can describe it easily and clearly.

Visceral nociceptors work a bit differently. That is not surprising, because the nociceptors that innervate the body's organs—the viscera—confront different threats from those facing skin, muscle, and bone. These nociceptors tend to be nonspecific, responding to a wider range of stimuli than the somatic nociceptors can manage—often, to stimuli around the periphery of a stimulus. And since the internal organs are continually expanding and contracting to execute their various functions, that means that visceral pain doesn't correlate in a clearly identifiable way to a specific instance of tissue damage; rather, it is perceived as "diffuse discomfort," in Farmer's phrase—uncomfortable but not so uncomfortable that your body can't tolerate performing those essential organ functions.

Moreover, in order for visceral nociceptors to become activated, a lot of stimulus at a high level of intensity is needed—these are high-threshold nerve endings, and it takes a long time for them to make their message heard. That also means that the sensation of pain can lag well behind the stimulus. All of this gives visceral pain its own particular quality—diffuse and hard to localize, quite different from the quality of somatic pain, just as chronic pain is quite different in quality from acute pain.

Where endometriosis is concerned, while the experience of pain is of course highly individual, those afflicted tend to describe the quality of the pain, using Farmer's terms, as visceral rather than somatic, chronic rather than acute.

For researchers of pain science and the brain, like Melissa Farmer, these differences in the quality of pain serve as a clue as to how and why a disease process like endometriosis evokes each of its varied symptoms of pain under varied circumstances. How, precisely, does endo get the CNS to respond as it does? Right now, says Farmer, the answer to that question is that "no one knows," but the research is ongoing. That research lies beyond the scope of this book, but any way you slice it, it is time to put to bed the notion that pain is just some primitive alarm system. Yes, it alerts the body to danger and in that sense serves a protective purpose, but it is also a complex web of inputs and outflows, of chemistry and electrical engineering and psychology, of connections and circuits. For the woman suffering from endo, the good news about this research is that it can lead to an understanding of how to break some of those connections and circuits and thus alleviate the disease's painful and damaging impacts.

In the meantime, we need to address the pain.

"MY NERVES ARE BURNING"

That's what patients tell us all the time. They describe sensations of burning, stabbing, tingling, numbness they feel "in the nerves" that crisscross the pelvic area, even travel down the legs, and for some, cause a shooting pain in the vagina or rectum. In the deepest and most intimate core of their bodies, these women feel like they are on fire.

Dr. Allyson Shrikhande is a physical medicine and rehabilitation specialist and an expert practitioner of a cutting-edge holistic treatment approach to pelvic pain and pelvic floor muscle dysfunction.* She is therefore well acquainted with the "fiery" pain these women describe. First, she says, because endo is "a proinflammatory state," the pelvic nerves of endo-afflicted women are, in Shrikhande's words, "swimming in an inflammatory soup." At the same time, the endo sufferer's abdominal and pelvic floor muscles tend to be in a chronic state of guarding against pain—the clenching action that Shrikhande says renders the muscles short, spastic, and weaker until, as she describes it, the muscles "essentially clamp down." As Amy adds, those clamped-down muscles "function poorly," compromising movement and stability.

Over time, that griplike tension in the muscles literally restricts blood flow in the immediate area and changes the pH balance there, which in turn "stimulates the inflammatory cascade" even further, adding to and "enriching" the inflammatory soup. The peripheral nociceptors in the pelvis, firing off like crazy as they sense all the damaging stimuli pouring out of this inflammatory cascade, go on overdrive; their input builds up and pushes the sensory messages up the spinal cord to the CNS and right up to the brain, which tells you that your pelvic area feels like it is on fire. A woman with endo, says Shrikhande, is in effect the target of "nociceptors firing aberrantly" and upregulating her CNS with every shot.

---

* She is also the chair of the Medical Education Committee for the International Pelvic Pain Society, among other credentials.

There is an additional factor at work as well: tissue trauma from endo lesions literally infiltrating the nociceptors of the PNS. You read back in chapter 1 about how endo cells grow denser with monthly hormonal fluctuations and how they create their own blood supply, essential for their survival. Those blood vessels are of course supplied with nerves, and as endo implants grow, the lesions also become innervated, and that innervation process follows the same pathway as the lesions—growing deeper, expanding outward, distorting the anatomy. Then somato-visceral and viscero-somatic cross-talk kicks in as well, spreading the pain from muscles and fascia to organ and back again, thereby amplifying the agony yet further. The nociceptors of the PNS fire off even more intently, and the pain just seems to spread.

A very likely prime mover of all this sensory information is the pudendal nerve—remember?—the main nerve of your pelvic floor at the body's core, the nerve that can play such a key role in painful sex. It is, says pelvic pain PT expert Stephanie Prendergast, a pioneering educator on the subject of pudendal neuralgia,[15] "a unique nerve," the only nerve in the entire body impacting organs and skeletal muscles equally. Affecting every sentient function from sex to sphincter—the urethra, genitals, rectum, the area between the genitals and anus, the buttocks, the thighs—the pudendal nerve can not only make sex too agonizing to bear, it often makes the sheer act of wearing pants feel like you've just walked into a searing flame.

That is what female pudendal neuralgia can feel like—yes, men get it too—and while it may be caused by a range of conditions and activities, enough endo patients suffer from it that it might almost be considered a by-product of the disease process itself. It follows the typically disastrous endo progression: lesions growing and expanding and distorting the anatomy, muscles and organs squeezing the nerves, nerves spreading the message of pain. But because its path is so "rigorous," as Amy describes it, an implant that's causing neural tension can become hyper-irritated in any number of ways—from the individual guarding against pain, possibly from the chronic inflammation of the body, maybe from getting sandwiched between ligaments.

Stephanie Prendergast's patients have described the various pains of pudendal neuralgia as like "a curling iron in the vagina," "a hot poker," "a pizza cutter inside me," "a Christmas tree in the butt," so when patients tell us that they feel their nerves are on fire and that the pain seems to spread everywhere, we know they are neither embroidering nor overdramatizing their pain or the scope of its reach.

Ice Massage to Cool Pudendal Neuralgia

Pudendal neuralgia is treatable, but it takes time and patience and the attention of a physical therapist specializing in pelvic pain. Here's a way, recommended by Amy, to cool the fire temporarily while you follow your individual treatment plan:

1. Freeze a Dixie cup full of water, then remove the top half of the cup to expose the ice.
2. Stand in the shower, as the ice will melt, and lift the leg on the side of your body that is in pain onto the rim of the shower or onto a stool.
3. Maintaining a circular motion so as to avoid ice burn, run the cup of ice along the path of pain from the tailbone to your vaginal opening along the crack in the buttocks.

SENSITIZATION AND THE
UPREGULATION OF THE CNS

Actually, the pain doesn't just "seem" to spread; it spreads. Also, it commonly gets worse; the pain can become amplified, more intense. The process is called sensitization; we both know it well, and we have mentioned it before, but to help explain it, we reached out to neurologist and pain physician Dr. Sheldon Jordan, a colleague who is a renowned expert in the subject.

Simply put, sensitization means that any original source of pain turns on additional pain pathways throughout the central nervous system—spinal cord and brain. As cells with receptors capable of responding to pain stimuli travel along a pathway, they recruit receptors in adjacent areas, mobilizing those receptors to respond to the pain stimuli as well. The more pathways recruited for your pain to travel along, the greater the number of receptors responding to the pain stimuli and the wider the expanse of the body the stimulus receptors occupy. The original source both intensifies and spreads. It hurts worse, and more of you hurts, and your bladder and bowel symptoms become even more distressing.

In time, the body becomes so sensitized that only the most minute stimulus is needed to experience pain. In one important study on pain management, researchers found that a "usually high-firing threshold" of the nociceptors that detect and carry the pain signal "decreases in the face of persistent pain."[16] In other words, it takes a lot less stimulus to send searing pain shooting through the body.

But for endo sufferers, what can really turn that pain into what seems like torture is that it tends to recur and recur and recur again—at least once a month, with each menstrual cycle, but from other provocations as well. What Dr. Jordan calls a "persistent and recurring pain stimulation" is what ignites the "capacity for in-creasing the sensitivity of the system," and it does so by effecting a change in the connectivity of the neurons carrying the message to the brain. These neurons—and the electrical signals in the brain that they spark—in effect "learn" or "remember" the frequent, re-peated stimulation; the next time the brain experiences that same stimulation, it responds faster and more potently. Recurring pain is thus something of a teaching tool: "The more a pain impulse travels through the system," says Dr. Jordan, "the more amplified it becomes."

Again, the amplification is characterized not only by a worsen-ing of the original source of pain but also by its widening scope—that is, the pain hurts more severely, and it hurts across a broader territory of the body. In time, what began as an entirely localized process can affect the entire central nervous system, with the re-sult that you can feel ever-worsening pain throughout your body, affecting your other organ systems—bladder, bowel, etc.—as well. Your CNS has been sensitized to be both more excited and more expansive in its excitability. That is the upregulation of the central nervous system in a painful and unhappy nutshell.

Think about years of pain stimuli and nerve excitation coursing through the central nervous system, speeding along the pathways of the spinal cord that ascend to the brain again and again, each trip "teaching" the pain to become more stimulated and the exci-tation more intense across more of the body. The result is an ever-widening geography of pain and an ever more excited response to stimulus till you quite possibly find yourself in the grip of a syndrome of total body pain and high-voltage sensitization.

There are also what Dr. Jordan refers to as the "secondary ef-fects" that occur as the individual tries to cope with her pain and worsening symptoms—in ways that unintentionally and indirectly amplify the sensitization yet further. Although these effects "have to do with the consequences of the original pain problem," says Dr. Jordan, they "can be involved in a very complicated feedback mechanism where the secondary factors make the original pain much worse." Ditto for your heightened bladder and bowel symptoms.

This vicious cycle typically starts when the pain—and the stress that results from it—makes it difficult to sleep. Failure to experience deep, restful sleep—slow-wave sleep, it is called—impairs the body's healing and regenerative mechanisms, depresses mood, and raises anxiety. This in turn leads to depression. Doing things becomes difficult, so the endo sufferer stops doing things, and stopping doing things worsens the pain. Dr. Jordan refers to this pattern of behavior as an escape-avoidance paradigm. It hurts to sit in a chair, so the endo sufferer stops sitting in a chair. It hurts to walk so she stays close to home. It hurts to have sex, so she stops that too. Pretty soon, her drive to avoid pain causes her to avoid just about all of life.

The motivation to take care of herself sinks. The woman finds it difficult to exercise and move her body. Moving the body is of course an important part of beating endo, and as Amy and Dr. Jordan point out, when you're not exercising, you are also not releasing the endorphins that are the body's natural pain fighters.

So instead, many women seek out prescription pain medication, which—while effective for some—also comes with a host of side effects and over time grows less effective (and therefore requires larger dosages). If the prescribed drug is an opiate, it is not only highly addictive, but as Amy notes and as Dr. Jordan articulates, it "actually sensitizes the pain pathways even further." Such drugs are not treating the CNS; they are simply masking symptoms.

In fact, in a cruel paradox, endo patients treated with opioids, says Jordan, experience even worse pain plus such symptoms as sleep disturbance, mood changes, inability to tolerate exercise, sensitivity to even light touch, and worsening bowel and bladder complaints. Nor does it end there.

As time passes—for example, the infamous twelve years between the onset of endo symptoms and its diagnosis—the pain that may have begun as a tiny dip into what Allyson Shrikhande described so vividly as "inflammatory soup" has so sensitized and upregulated the entire CNS that several things happen:

First, as noted, the body has learned the pain lesson so well that only the most minute stimulus is needed to cause the pain. A key research study on pain management has pointed out that the "usually high-firing threshold" of the nociceptors that detect and carry the pain signal "decreases in the face of persistent pain."[17] It just takes a lot less stimulus to send searing pain shooting through the body.

Second, the pain really is everywhere. The buildup of sensory data in the brain's cortex, which maps the body, spills over the map's borders into areas nowhere near the original source of pain, having recruited so many adjacent areas around the original pathways that what started as a localized nerve irritation has become an all-systems disaster.

Third, the viscero-somatic and somato-visceral cross-talk that pain stimuli may invoke ups the ante even further, so that the stimulation of pain becomes an almost spontaneous occurrence. Years of endo have rendered your pain a reaction so "built in" to your CNS that the slightest whisper of almost any kind of stimulus sets off your entire body. Your central nervous system is effectively firing on its own.

That is not how we want any woman to live.

A STRATEGY FOR BEATING ENDO:
DESENSITIZATION/DOWNREGULATION

The more pain you have, the worse your pain is and the more widely you feel both the pain and your symptoms: This is a phenomenon we see in just about every realm of healthcare. The patient arriving for a knee replacement surgery is asked to fill out a body map showing exactly where he or she feels pain. The patient whose body map shows pain only on the knee about to be replaced will most likely sail through the surgery, leave the hospital quickly, require fewer opioids during recovery, and heal faster. The patient whose map shows pain in the knee about to be replaced *and* in the other knee, in the shoulder, the neck, the hip, the feet—you get the picture—is likely to "perform" in precisely the opposite way, with a long hospital stay, a difficult recovery, lots of painkillers, and slow healing. That is a patient whose CNS has become globally sensitized, and replacing a bum knee will not be sufficient to bring him or her to health. All it does is lift one hand off the stove, and that's just not enough.

For the endo patient overburdened by years of this CNS sensitization, the widening pain is augmented by the full panoply of Dr. Jordan's "secondary effects." These patients are exhausted from living with a chronic inflammatory process, from lack of sleep, and from the tiring process of repeating the same symptoms over and over to doctor after doctor. In many cases, they have been dismissed by the "experts" or told their disease is in their heads or is something they "just have to live with." Their lives have been narrowed, their sex lives diminished, their work lives put on hold, their relationships limited—so they are quite naturally anxious and depressed, and, as we have seen, anxiety and depression are engines of the sensitization of the central nervous system. There is a psychological aspect to what happens in the CNS, and there is a mental-health price to pay for what endo does to the CNS.

An endo patient's susceptibility to sensitization of the CNS is also linked to her susceptibility to autoimmune diseases. In an autoimmune disorder, as the body's immune system attacks itself, one aberrant condition creates a path to another, producing a cascade of damaging effects. A freaked-out central nervous system is not only a body in pain, it can also be the starting gun that sets off other morbidities—and that too raises the stakes of an endo patient's suffering.

When the central nervous system has become its own pain generator, taking one hand off the stove won't work. You must take them all off. You must calm your ramped-up CNS globally, peeling back one layer of the onion after another after another till the onion is no longer an onion. Sheldon Jordan puts it this way: "Desensitization has to precede" any other interventions. And desensitization—achieved by downregulating your central nervous system—is the bedrock of beating endo.

A not atypical patient for both of us is a woman who remembers having had sufficiently bad cramps as a young girl that she typically missed a day of school once a month, or spent hours in the school nurse's office, or both. Her bladder and gastrointestinal tract were also not functioning well, and a worried parent took her to one specialist after another in what we've called "misdiagnosis roulette." Her musculoskeletal system became increasingly affected—tightened—as the years went by, and she was more tired in college and in her twenties than most of her friends. Depressed too, as her co-conditions accumulated and her burning CNS spun her downward. Maybe the patient had ablation surgery, felt a bit better for a time, but as the pain returned found herself turning more and more to the opioids prescribed for post-surgery. They helped, briefly, with the "burning nerves" in her pelvis and the joint pain she can't shake and the migraines. But the relief did not last, and now, feeling at the end of her rope, she is wondering if she shouldn't just go ahead with a hysterectomy . . .*

This "typical" patient, fictional though she is, is not an anomaly. We can number in the thousands patients who fit the description perfectly. By the time they come to us, the conditions that could have been—should have been—addressed from the start have spiraled out of control. It is why Iris is so intent on identifying endo in teens or adolescents and beginning the downregulation then—before the spiral ever starts. Wherever you "fit" in that story of our typical patient, the time to start your desensitizing/downregulating is now. A downregulated system is the prerequisite to letting yourself heal.

HERNIAS: ANOTHER SOURCE OF NERVE PAIN

In addition, women with endo sometimes also present with hernias, which are defects in the fascia. The four most common in the abdomino-pelvic region are inguinal, obturator, femoral, and umbilical. Allyson tells us that "given the referred pain patterns, they can be difficult to diagnose and distinguish on history and exam alone. The inguinal, obturator, and femoral hernias can

---

* Once more: The notion that hysterectomy is a treatment for endometriosis is a myth—and a pernicious one.

cause groin discomfort that hurts worse with lifting, straining, and standing." Inguinal hernias can cause pain in the ilioinguinal nerve along the inguinal canal—which translates into pain in the lower part of the abdominal wall—and into the pelvic floor muscles. "The patient can describe a vague, dull, deep ache or a burning, knifelike, stabbing sensation if the nerve is significantly involved," says Shrikhande. It is why Iris always checks for hernias during an initial consultation and, helped by preoperative imaging, looks for them during surgery.

COMING TO GRIPS WITH YOUR
UPREGULATED CNS

We've already presented in some detail one of the most essential methods for calming your central nervous system: physical therapy. All of the Basic Six exercises we outlined on pages 69 to 74—and certainly the first two, conscious breathing and the pelvic drop—are excellent ways to cool the CNS at any time. And a qualified physical therapist, in hands-on sessions, can offer an array of effective techniques for addressing each of the conditions that have raised the temperature of your central nervous system.

In addition, there is a range of medical treatments that can help downregulate the CNS, including certain medications, and there are other modalities that may *complement* the approaches we discuss throughout this book, but of course all such treatments should be administered by qualified professional practitioners. And in no way should any of them supplant the peeling back of one co-condition after another that we put forth in the pages that follow.

Other Treatments and Modalities

We believe all the following treatments and modalities can be effective in addressing an upregulated CNS if applied properly and monitored by a qualified healthcare provider. By "applied properly," we mean, for example, ensuring that you are on the right medication dosage for treating the CNS sensitization; this means starting slowly and possibly taking weeks or months of increasing the dose till you reach the therapeutic level, which is when effectiveness begins to kick in. Obviously, that also means choosing a doctor who understands how to treat the CNS. Here are just some of the more common treatments and modalities your healthcare provider may suggest to you to address an up-regulated CNS, but this is by no means a complete list.

Medications for chronic sensitization: Lyrica, Neurontin
Medications for generalized pain: Cymbalta, Savella
Local suppositories compounded of Valium and/or baclofen once or twice a day
Pelvic sympathetic block
Injections for pelvic floor dysfunction by a trained specialist
CBD (cannabidiol)
Some nutraceuticals, especially curcumin (unless you have painful bladder syndrome)

We have said from the beginning of this book that we would be offering a multimodal approach to beating endo—a protocol that would touch on all aspects of the disease condition. It's no accident, after all, that Amy calls her business Beyond Basics Physical Therapy and relies on reaching out to established experts in nutrition, acupuncture, meditation and mindfulness, yoga, and many more disciplines. Amy finds acupuncture particularly helpful for her patients in downregulating the central nervous system, increasing blood flow, calming trigger points, and optimizing bladder and bowel function. There is no single magic bullet for this disease (or for most diseases), so the aim is to optimize your body's functioning in as many ways as possible so that it can fight your endo while giving you the best possible quality of life.

It is to that end—the optimization of your body's functioning—that we're recommending three main approaches you can *undertake on your own*—in addition to and along with proper treatment of your endo disease under the guidance of an endometriosis specialist and a physical therapist. Each approach requires making changes in a fundamental category of lifestyle behavior, and each category offers numerous choices among varied practices and techniques. The categories are nutrition—since eating is essential, nutrition is the first layer of the onion; environment—the things you surround yourself with in your daily life; and mindfulness—what you can do to heal and restore the hardware of the brain and thereby cool the central nervous system.

The methods we will offer for making these changes are all simply tools of healthy living for just about everyone and for the course of a lifetime. Yet we are both aware that there is a very human tendency to regard the recommended practices as chores we'd prefer to avoid. We know because we've been there. We've been reluctant to give up things we think we love and to take on responsibilities that at first can seem tedious and burdensome. That's one reason we stated early on in this book that beating endo would require commitment.

The key to making and maintaining that commitment is to find, among all the techniques and practices of the next three chapters, the ones that work for you. Those are the ones you will stick to, so it is well worth it to fill your individual toolbox with a sliding scale of tools you know you will use. Iris insists that "everyone has a something they can stick to." And she adds that "what's right for your sister may not be right for you, so you need to find your own something."

We did. It took a bit of doing, particularly in finding a way to chill out and cool down our central nervous systems, but we each found the right tool:

Amy had always thought meditation practice sounded like a wonderful way to become more mindful and calm the CNS. But the minute she sat down in a quiet place and tried to empty her brain, it filled up with all the projects going on at work, all the things on her plate at home, and all the appointments on her calendar for the next day. What worked instead was a hike in the woods. Walking away, into a totally different environment, pushed appointments and projects right out of her head and focused her brain instead on the terrain she was passing through, the sounds of the forest, the single need to put one foot after another—in short, awareness of the present moment, the perfect calming mechanism for a revved-up state of mind. When city life makes a woods walk impossible, Amy gets a similar effect in an exercise regimen in which she focuses on frequency and duration, not on the kind of intensity that proved so detrimental to endo patient Taylor back in chapter 2. An athlete in school and a veteran skier and snowboarder who is at home in natural places, Amy finds physical activity, especially in the open air, a commitment to be relished.

For Iris, the tool is yoga capped by an ocean swim, and doing both regularly has been transformative. As a doctor—not to mention as a wife and mother—her phone rings and pings a lot: Patients reach her at all hours, emergencies happen, and the thinking and researching and studying that are essential to her work are ongoing. There is scant downtime for the brain and less than that for the body. But there are no cell phones in yoga class, where she prefers Hot Vinyasa in which each movement is linked to a breath in the flow from one pose to the next. For Iris, this is restorative, releasing the brain, easing the body, and when both are in sync, providing inner peace. After that, the ocean swim feels like a body-brain dessert.

ENDO AND NUTRITION

We know: It really doesn't seem fair. As if it weren't enough, if you are a woman with endo, you are saddled with uncomfortable, distressing, limiting pains and dysfunctions. Now, on top of it all, we're telling you to give up Ben & Jerry's Coffee Toffee Bar Crunch forever?

You're right—it's not fair. But the reality is this: What you eat can either fuel your endo pain or help diminish it. So think of the nutritional strategies that follow as empowering rather than depriving. The choices you make about what you eat can serve as a powerful weapon in beating the disease.

That weapon is solely in your hands, for obviously everybody eats, and everybody must eat to stay alive. Digestion is the process by which the body makes all that happen; it carries out the work of creating the acids and enzymes that break down the food and get it absorbed into our system. That means that how and how well digestion functions is essential to how well we live—and to how well we feel. And endo, of course, can complicate that function, especially where certain foods are concerned.

A core problem, unfortunately, is that the standard Western diet that we have been eating all our lives sets a high hurdle for endo to overcome. Simply put, the foods the standard diet favors are decidedly pro-inflammatory, and if it has been your primary diet for any length of time, inflammation is most likely already systemic within you. That systemic inflammation, the precursor to many serious diseases, may already be affecting your well-being in various additional ways over and above the disease of endometriosis, for inflammation can adversely impact bones and skin, can irritate your gastrointestinal tract, burden your sleep, affect your ability to maintain a healthy weight, weaken your gums, and bring on depression—in addition to potentially contributing to heart disease, cancer, and lung problems. Add in the fact that endometriosis is an inflammatory process with many characteristics of an autoimmune disease, and the systemic inflammation within you is something you will want to counter. As this chapter sets forth, you can do so both by avoiding many of the foods that have probably been part of your own standard, contemporary Western diet and by seeking out different foods instead.

But that isn't all that the standard Western diet does to women with endo. It also fails to supply them with enough of the right prebiotics, the indigestible plant fibers that feed the probiotics, which are the microbes within the gut that stimulate good digestion. Insufficient prebiotics means a less diverse and less healthy microbial environment in the colon—bad bacteria in the gut—outweighing the power of the good probiotics. "Poor bacterial health in the colon," notes nutritionist Jessica Drummond, with whom we consulted in some depth for the writing of this chapter, "is a physical stressor that can lead to hormonal imbalances, including estrogen dominance and dis-regulated stress hormone and insulin levels." Removing certain foods from your diet and adding others can help restore the balance.

In addition, the secondary digestive symptoms that women with endo often suffer—irritable bowel syndrome or a range of colon issues—can exacerbate the situation by upregulating the nervous system further. And all of this is amplified by the pain that burdens so many endo patients, especially chronic pain, because pain is an agent of depletion; it consumes the biochemical energy needed to get the job of digestion done. The bottom line for going up against all of these effects of endo—inflammation, a less than optimal gut microbiome, and an upregulated central nervous system—is that changing what and how you eat can mitigate all of these situations. Doing so is downright essential for women with endo.

You have no doubt heard this before. You've read it in these pages as well, as we have already noted a number of caveats about certain kinds of foods earlier in this book. We have repeatedly noted the benefits of an anti-inflammatory diet; in chapter 4, we advocated a specifically low-acid, low-potassium diet for women with bladder issues; and in chapter 5 we discussed specific foods to be avoided and others to be embraced to calm down a troubled GI tract. We continue to recommend an anti-inflammatory diet as beneficial for women with endo, coupled with a low-acid, low-potassium approach to eating for those with bladder issues. In general, we can say that a primarily organic plan of nutrition that avoids major inflammation sensitivities and that provides sufficient nutrients and energy is the way to go. While we might not call this an "endo diet," an anti-inflammatory way of eating—indeed, an anti-inflammatory way of *living*—is essential for any woman with endo.

In fact, as we don't have to assert at this point, the impact of endo's varied symptoms is so individual, and its consequences are so diffuse throughout the body and in a way so "distant" from the disease *per se*, that the idea of a single "endo diet" makes no sense. What may alleviate the symptoms of a co-condition in you may not work at all against the same co-condition in another woman. Nor is every woman's central nervous system sensitized to the same degree or in the same way. So the foods one endo patient avoids like the plague may be another endo patient's harmless indulgence. The human digestive system, in other words, is very nearly as individual as human fingerprints. But what we can tell you in this chapter is what you ought to consider overall as you set out to create your own "diet"—the kinds of foods and an approach to eating that can not only mitigate your particular symptoms but keep you healthy and enable you to thrive.

Almost inevitably, that is going to mean changing your nutrition habits, and we will offer some tips on the practical issues involved in proceeding to do that—where to find the information you need, why and where to get the assistance that may make it all more understandable and easier. We'll suggest too that changing your nutrition may also mean changing how you eat—your eating behavior. But we begin with our major recommendation—that is, the focus on alleviating inflammation through what you eat and what you avoid eating.

AN ANTI-INFLAMMATORY WAY OF EATING

We know that inflammation is the body's protective response to harmful stimuli or damaged cells or irritants. It is the marshaling of a range of defense mechanisms that spark immune system reactions. The problem is that the body's immune system never goes off duty, and that is why Iris's succinct argument for avoiding pro-inflammatory foods is so powerful: "If you have endo, you *already have* inflammation. Pro-inflammatory foods tip the scales." When that happens, the immune system can get stuck in a constant defensive mode—chronic inflammation.

So the essential first step is to avoid pro-inflammatory categories of food, including dairy, gluten, soy, sugar, and artificial sweeteners, all of which, by the way, are found in Coffee Toffee Bar Crunch and most other ice creams. Avoid these "top five" food categories.

Keep in mind that, unlike the environmental pollutants we'll discuss in the next chapter—which more or less harm you slowly, over time—food represents a pretty direct and quick hit. The journey from ingestion through the digestive tract to absorption into the body's blood, tissue, muscles, and so on is uncomplicated and moves at a fairly swift pace. This is one reason you may already know that certain foods, especially those in the top five pro-inflammatory categories, affect you in certain ways.

In addition to the top five, avoid as much as possible foods that are artificially processed; they too can provoke inflammatory responses. By "artificially processed," we mean foods that have been so broken down and modified that they bear little relation, if any, to the original form of the food they claim to be. Potato chips versus the potato, for example. "Convenience" meals: Just warm up the package on the stove, and dinner is ready to ingest. Junk food snacks, of course. "Lunch meats" and deli meats, pre-packaged and cured, from cheap baloney to the high-priced *soprassata* imported from Italy. Add to these any vegetables and fruits that have only grown at all because they were sprayed with pesticides or that have been preserved over the course of a long truck ride thanks to para-bens: These also qualify as "processed."*

Does this mean that everything in each of the five major pro-inflammatory sensitivities is a no-no forever? Or are there specific foods a woman with endo should avoid or, conversely, might ben-efit from focusing on?

The only way to figure that out is through trial and error. You can formalize the process by noting what you eat and how you react to each food or combination of foods; you probably know the main culprits that inflame your system already. Or focus on each one of the five categories at a time in your own experiment—again: dairy, gluten, soy, sugar, and artificial sweeteners. Try cutting out the entire category for a set period; if that proves to be too limiting for you, then add back one food at a time to see your reaction.

Amy once gave up dairy as an experiment to see if and how it might affect her. She eliminated all dairy foods from her diet entirely for two weeks, then began adding back one dairy item at a time to assess her response. Her body's feedback, she says, was fast and clear; within a month, she had learned a lot about what to avoid and what she could happily and healthily continue to eat. You can do the same; a month isn't a terribly long time to experi-ment on something.

The other four of the top five inflammatory categories present slower trial-and-error processes; their effects tend to be tougher to analyze and take longer to become manifest. But a sensible amount of self-testing might be worth your while before you seek out a nutritionist to work with for the longer term. Our preeminent rec-ommendation as you set out to change what and how you eat is

---

* Frozen fruits and vegetables are exceptions; they are frozen at harvest and main-tain their quality and plenty of their nutritional value.

that you do just that—find a nutritionist who can help you plan the right tests, evaluate the responses, and keep you as healthy as possible as the two of you figure out what works and what doesn't during the trial-and-error period.

Why do we recommend professional expertise? The truth is that where beating endo is concerned, "it is less about food than about how each individual's digestion is functioning" in the words of Jessica Drummond, noted and quoted earlier in this chapter. Jessica is the founder of the Integrative Women's Health Institute; she is also a world-renowned pioneer in the creation of nutrition disciplines for women with pelvic health issues. While steering clear of the five main sensitivities for inflammation is a good start, Jessica suggests there is much more to consider when it comes to beating endo.

DIGESTIVE FUNCTION

Which foods do you tolerate well, and which give you trouble? How do you eat—on the way to work out of a cardboard container, seated and relaxed so that you can chew your food slowly and well and create adequate juices for the digestive process, *en route* to the gym, or maybe standing up waiting for a text to arrive? How much and how well do you chew your food? What is the source of the foods you eat? Is organic food or "high-quality" food financially out of your reach? Do you like to cook, take the time to cook, find cooking a chore and a bore? All of this can affect your digestive function—that is, how well your system creates the juices and enzymes that break down what you've eaten so that it is absorbed into the body as fuel to power and sustain the life you live.

Genetic predisposition also affects digestive function, and as we all know, there's not much you can do about what you "inherited" in your genes. Take as an example people with blood type O; as Jessica explains, they commonly have higher levels of stomach acid and can easily digest fats and proteins. That means that they can thrive on a nutrition plan much like that of the paleo diet, which embraces animal proteins, fish and seafood, fresh fruits and vegetables, eggs, nuts, and seeds. It also means that they are going to be a lot less happy eating grains. People with other blood types, however, do better on a plant-based diet. On the other hand, Drummond notes, "if you have blood type O but have had endo and chronic pain for fifteen years," that could diminish your levels of stomach acid despite your genetic inheritance. In turn, Jessica adds, that might necessitate moving away from "a nutrition plan that includes higher amounts of animal protein until you make nutrition and lifestyle changes to restore the optimal functioning of your stomach acid and other digestive juices."

The bottom line is that human beings are too individual—and their digestive functions too distinctive—for us or anybody to issue a list of absolute commandments, even absolute recommendations that all endo patients should follow. Amy notes that even the simplest "general rule" can become highly specific, depending on the circumstances. For example, while nuts like almonds are anti-inflammatory stalwarts—with their omega fatty acids, unsaturated fats, and fiber also contributing to heart health—eating too many of them turns them pro-inflammatory. What constitutes "too many" almonds? A nutritionist can help you find your limit.

Probably the first thing a nutritionist can help you with is an understanding of who you are as an eater—your eating profile, so to say. You want to understand the characteristics of your own digestive function, to find out, as best you can, about your genetic digestive "inheritance," and to note the character and quality of the foods available to you. You also need to assess frankly your overall stress level. These considerations define you as an eater and will affect your eating behavior, which will in turn affect your endo symptoms. Creating such a profile shows you the boundaries and directions within which you can create a nutrition plan that will help you beat endo.

YOUR ENDO NUTRITION PLAN

We said "no absolutes," but for endo sufferers, some really really strong recommendations are in order. By all means, remove from your diet, to the greatest extent possible, those five inflammatory sensitivities: dairy, gluten, soy, sugar, and artificial sweeteners. Where dairy is concerned, Jessica Drummond suggests that women with endo should just "eliminate it—long term." Avoid the aforementioned processed foods as well; they too can trigger inflammation. If you suspect you are sensitive to eggs, eliminate them too.

How do you stop eating foods you've eaten your entire life? There is no trick to it: Just stop eating them. Reject them, politely, if they are offered to you. Look right past them on the menu at your favorite restaurant or in the grocery store. Today there are so many delicious alternatives that it's easy to find substitutes that will satisfy—from nut milks to coconut yogurt to vegan ice cream to non-grain-based flours like almond and chickpea.

Then, set a long-term goal of eating from eight to ten servings of organic vegetables every day. A single serving of cooked vegetables means about half a cup; a serving of raw vegetables is conceivably twice that: one cup. So even as many as ten servings of vegetables do not represent excessive abundance for a day's intake. Figure it as about the equivalent of one and a half to two heaping platefuls of pasta. The ultimate aim is to ensure that your diet is plant-based, but start slowly, and start with cooked vegetables—blended soups are a great beginning—because raw vegetables are harder to digest. If your current diet consists of just one or two vegetable servings a day, take a good while to meet the eight-to-ten-a-day goal—four, five, six months if needed. Don't jump there at once on the theory that the sooner you hit the mark, the better you'll feel. On the contrary: You want to work your way up, giving your digestive system time to adjust and letting your central nervous system downregulate along the way.

Leafy green vegetables are perfect choices for daily vegetable servings. Lettuce, kale, spinach, parsley, endive, arugula, bok choy, Swiss chard, and the like have all been called "powerfoods" because they are so full of nutrients, because you can eat them cooked or raw (but remember, start with cooked), and because they are distinctly flavorful. All of those factors make the leafy greens a bonanza for creative chefs as well as for nutritionists.

Jessica reminds us that among green vegetables, the crucifers are particularly beneficial for women with endo because they help metabolize the excess estrogen in their systems. Crucifers—the word means "cross-bearer"—are distinguished by their flowers: typically four in number, arranged diagonally, like a cross. In addition to the kale, arugula, Swiss chard, and bok choy noted above, they include broccoli, Brussels sprouts, cabbage, and cauliflower.

Jessica also cautions readers to exercise care with the nightshade vegetables—tomatoes, potatoes, peppers, zucchini, and eggplant—because of endo's autoimmune qualities. Nightshades can trigger an inflammatory response that might ignite the immune system, so test carefully before embracing these vegetables.

Along the way, as you work your way up to the eight-to-ten veggie servings a day—and once you've achieved the goal as well, of course—make sure that 30 percent of your diet consists of healthy fats. Everyone needs a reasonable amount of fat. Certainly every woman does, and most certainly every woman with endo does because, by definition, she will have low levels of progesterone along with her high levels of estrogen. It is true that fat is, as Jessica puts it, "a precursor to *all* hormones," but the woman with endo needs to build up her progesterone, and that "reasonable" 30 percent of your diet in healthy fats is therefore essential.

What healthy fats are we talking about? Avocados, of course; olive oil and coconut oil; nuts and seeds that have been soaked first (see sidebar); fatty fish like salmon, tuna, anchovies, herring—all wild-caught; eggs, if you can tolerate them; and, unless you suffer from painful bladder syndrome, for which it can be an irritant, let us not forget dark chocolate.* All qualify as healthy fats.

Why Soak Nuts and Seeds?

Dry seeds—particularly chia, flax, hemp, and pumpkin seeds—contain hard-to-digest enzyme inhibitors in large amounts. Soaking them neutralizes the enzymes, effectively igniting the germination process—you can sometimes see the sprouting—which your digestive system forestalls. Any nuts you eat regularly should be soaked as well.

---

* As defined by the Food and Drug Administration, dark chocolate contains a minimum of 35 percent cacao beans; Amy says "healthy dark chocolate" really contains 70 percent cacao beans.

What about protein? It is of course an essential building block
of the body and therefore should be an essential part of any nutrition plan. On an endo nutrition plan, it should also be easily
digestible—if beans are your preferred protein, be sure they have
been soaked and are cooked slowly—and should be from as clean a
source as possible, whether plant-based or animal-based. Those requirements probably mean that your protein should be sourced as
locally as possible because local means a shorter distance between
the origin of the food—farm, body of water, woods (for the hunters
among you), chicken coop—and your table. For plant-based foods,
defining the cleanest source may also mean "certified organic." For
poultry, it typically means free-range birds that were never fed antibiotics and are certified organic. For beef, it means grass-fed and
certified organic. For fish, it can mean certified as caught wild in
"cleaner" waters and under sustainable-fishing practices.

Those are tall orders, and there's no doubt that these requirements can raise the price of food. The fertilizers and pesticides
and supplements developed for "industrial agriculture" have been
aimed at creating "product" quickly and efficiently and getting it
to your supermarket as fast as possible. "Clean" or organic farm-
ing relies not on chemicals but on manual labor and on such applied techniques as crop rotation—not as easy, not as cheap, not as
fast. Also, organic food just tends to grow slowly. As do grass-fed
cattle. And heading out to catch wild fish takes a lot longer than
harvesting them right at the fish farm. For those and other reasons, slower-to-harvest foods cost more; time is money, after all.

In addition, harvested organic agricultural yields are typically
shipped separately from those of major agricultural enterprises and,
being smaller, cost more to handle and ship. It all adds up. Even in
growing season, when these foods can typically be purchased fairly
directly—that is, not too far from home at a local farmers market,

at fairs, at shops catering to customers concerned about the quality of what they eat—they are still likely to be costlier than more "convenient" foods. It will be up to you to determine whether their benefits to your health are worth the price.

Grains present a different kind of problem. They can spark an inflammatory response that impedes the absorption of amino acids, essential for boosting the immune system. Given endo's autoimmune characteristics, this makes consuming grains a tricky issue. Moreover, most grains sold today are "refined," which means they have been stripped of their nutrient-rich properties, so endo sufferers who want to keep grains in their diet should make sure they are choosing whole grains.

And there *are* potential benefits for keeping such whole grains in the diet, especially for those endo patients who exercise frequently and may be energy-depleted. For these women, grains like quinoa, millet, and brown rice can be beneficial overall and a helpful addition to the diet. This makes grains a bit like eggs—that is, a double-edged sword. Your best bet is to test your tolerance under the guidance of a nutritionist.

THE PRACTICALITIES

Making changes to the way you eat—and possibly to the way your family eats—is no small matter. Where do you start? Again, we recommend finding a nutritionist to help you. Indeed, we both think it is almost as important to find that practitioner as it is to find the right doctor or physical therapist. How to find the right one? By all means, start at the Integrative Women's Health Institute website— www.integrativewomenshealthinstitute.com. That is the website of Jessica Drummond's organization, and the first place to look there is in the provider directory, which contains a list of practitioners, their qualifications, a description of their specialty, and contact information. Many of the nutritionists in the site's directory see patients virtually and will consult over the phone, even if they're not in your area. Another resource is the Institute for Functional Medicine, at www.ifm.org. Unlike traditional Western medicine in which specialists are siloed in their individual fields, functional medicine, aimed squarely at complex chronic disease, begins from an "analysis of common underlying pathways that interact to produce disease and dysfunction," according to its medical textbook, and aims at a personalized model of treatment. Whether or not they are nutrition specialists, functional medicine practitioners think in terms of cause and effect in the interconnections among the various bodily systems. They've made the paradigm shift from matching symptoms to a pathology to exploring the underlying processes and working to fix the impaired function. Both the Integrative Women's Health Institute and the Institute for Functional Medicine have trained practitioners all over the world, and both websites offer ongoing education, blogs or podcasts, and other resources.

Among them, Jessica recommended to us and we are recommending unreservedly to you the website Nourishing Meals, www.nourishingmeals.com. It is mostly veggie-oriented, and its recipes are as varied and creative as they are excellent—especially for blended soups, notes Jessica—and it is an easy-to-get-around, highly informative, neatly intuitive website as well.

We are also happy to recommend *Nutrition for Relieving Pelvic Pain: Fueling the Patient/Practitioner Healing Partnership*, the cookbook of the Integrative Women's Health Network, authored by Jessica Drummond and the Institute's recipe designers, and published in January 2019.

Your new way of eating is not a free pass to stop reading the ingredients lists on food packages. In fact, you may have to look particularly carefully for "hidden" ingredients down the list. Vegans will have to check for additives like casein, for glaze on sweet items, even for honey. Soy avoiders should check if their vegetable oil is actually soybean oil, and so forth. Yes, standing there squinting at small-type lists is a bit of a chore, but in time, it becomes automatic—especially if your new way of eating has brought some relief to your symptoms. And, as we'll be telling you more about in the very next chapter, you have a powerful ally for food shopping in the website of the Environmental Working Group—www.ewg.org.

HOW YOU EAT

Stress gets blamed for a lot of things, and where digestion is concerned, it takes a well-deserved big hit, as its effects are no picnic, to put it mildly. An upregulated CNS can contract the digestive muscles, wrench the colon into a twist, and above all put the brakes on your gut's production of digestive acids and therefore on your digestive system's ability to break down foods properly. So the "mood" you bring to the breakfast nook, the lunchroom, or the dinner table—the extent to which you have cooled your CNS or failed to do so—can cause not just pain and discomfort but functional damage as well.

Another thing to consider is not only what and how you eat, but also what you drink. We recommend against endo sufferers consuming alcohol for a couple of reasons. One is because it is a physical stressor; it stimulates the HPA (hypothalamic pituitary adrenal) axis, which is the body's central stress response system. Another reason is that it can be high in sugar, and sugar generates inflammation in the body. (It is also a real no-no if you have painful bladder syndrome.) On the other hand, if you have come to the table in a relaxed way, a glass of organic wine *with* food just might add to the relaxed feeling, in the wine drinker's mind anyway. Sugary alcoholic drinks—frozen margaritas come to mind—are definitely beyond the pale, as are the brown spirits like rum, whiskey, and bourbon. If it's a festive occasion and you feel a drink will help you to de-stress and relax a bit, mix a shot of tequila with some lime, or enjoy a glass of wine, or sip a vodka with soda water and lemon. All that said, if you have painful bladder syndrome, we recommend forgoing alcohol (and carbonated drinks) and the citrus fruits to flavor them entirely.

And don't forget to chew your food well. Gulping down food without chewing it sufficiently burdens the digestive system; that food needs to get chopped up and ground down, and it takes teeth to do it. As Jessica Drummond likes to say, "There are no teeth in the stomach." They are all in your mouth, and putting them to work is extremely important to getting the nutrition you need.

Way back in the late nineteenth and early twentieth centuries, an American food enthusiast named Horace Fletcher (1849–1919) advocated chewing your food no fewer than thirty-five and as many as one hundred times before swallowing. It came to be known as "Fletcherizing" your food, and it's worth keeping in mind. "Nature will castigate those who don't masticate," Horace Fletcher was famous for saying. It is funny to us now, and Fletcherization is easy to deride, but "The Great Masticator," as he was called, may yet have the last laugh. Endo sufferers would do well to follow the spirit, if not necessarily the letter, of Fletcher's preaching.

Cool your mind and adjust your mood, then settle down to a meal, relax, eat healthy and hearty food, and chew it well.

And whatever you do, try not to feel deprived. The world of

food is so vast and varied, and we live in a time of so much interest in so many forms of healthy eating that it really is very easy indeed to focus on the positive. In your kitchen, where you rule over ingredients, methods, and menus, you can be as creative as you like. Recipes abound—on Instagram, in food blogs, in cookbooks. Embrace the nutritional guidelines recommended for endo sufferers and be inspired—by your imagination, your creativity, your sense of adventure, and your sense of taste.

ENDO AND YOUR ENVIRONMENT

That 1992 research study we noted in chapter 1—made possible by Mary Lou Ballweg and the Endometriosis Association—did more than confirm the connection between dioxin exposure and endometriosis. The study also alerted us to the fact that there are substances in common use, predominantly synthetic chemical substances, that can have an adverse impact on our bodies. For endo sufferers in particular, the study specifically pointed out the potential of these substances to alter hormonal levels.

"Endocrine disruptors" is the term applied to these chemicals because that is exactly what they do: They upend, distort, and impede the way the endocrine system secretes hormones into the bloodstream. They imitate hormones in the body, interfere with hormonal signals, transform a particular hormone into an entirely different hormone, bind themselves to essential hormones, and build up in the organs that create hormones, among other disruptions. They are often pseudo-estrogens; that means they trick the body into recognizing them as estrogen and thus trigger the same effects as real estrogen would. There is even research exploring whether certain chemical endocrine disruptors might be a risk factor for developing endometriosis.

The bottom line is that chemicals that can potentially harm you and intensify your pain are present in many standard, everyday products you have in your home, or that you come into contact with in the course of your day, or that you buy for your personal use. Over time, if their presence in your life is extensive or persistent, they can have an adverse impact on your health and on your ability to fight your endo. So part of our plan for beating endo is to help you learn about the chemicals in the products you use; as throughout this book, education is the first armament empowering better, more informed choices for your health.

Here's one way to think about it: It isn't enough to focus solely on the quality and source of the food we buy. We also have to consider the pan we cook it in and the containers we store it in. For example, if you buy yourself a nice gluten-free, dairy-free meal but it is packaged in plastic, you might well be taking in some of those aforementioned endocrine disruptors as well as setting off an inflammatory response in your body. That would sort of cancel out some of the good you counted on with your choice of food. The simple solution is to buy a glass food container for your next meal and to repurpose the plastic container into a receptacle for nails and screws and stash it in the garage. A little effort, to be sure, but doable.

Indeed, there is very good news about dealing with risks in your environments, for not only is there a wealth of knowledge about how to identify and avoid these endocrine disruptors *and* about what to use instead, but the knowledge is available literally at your fingertips via the internet. And there is that one website we mentioned briefly, Iris's all-time favorite on which she draws for keeping both her family and her patients healthy, that of the Environmental Working Group, at www.ewg.org—a portal into instant answers, drawn from years of ongoing, in-depth research, to just about any question you have. In other words, for this change in lifestyle behavior, there is help aplenty.

If it sounds like there may be a lot of information to take in, never fear. Ease into the change. Take one step at a time and let yourself experiment until you find the substitute, workaround, or solution that both works for you and makes you feel good.

Let's begin by understanding what's at stake here for endo sufferers.

THE RISK

A 2016 research study[18] focused on two sets of chemical toxins that can be particularly harmful to endo sufferers. The study calls these "persistent chemicals" and "nonpersistent chemicals," which doesn't leave much of an escape route. Both groups can be toxic, but the first group includes toxins that don't break down easily and persist in our environment though outlawed long ago. They're referred to as POPs, persistent organic pollutants, and they include dioxins, perhaps the *primo* endocrine disruptors of all time. Dioxins in turn belong to a group of substances known as organochlorines, which are found everywhere on earth, and although production of dioxin was banned in 2001, and another organochlorine, PCBs (polychlorinated biphenyls), was banned in 1978, these toxins may still affect us. In fact, while production of dioxin is now illegal, and while its natural production through forest fires or the burning of trash is way down, some dioxin releases from decades ago are still around to trip us up.

Actually, we get it primarily in food, specifically from the fat content in meat and dairy foods. Beef, pork, poultry, and eggs are the main sources, and the bad news is that all dairy products *may* contain dioxins handed down through the generations from the time the chemical was widely in use. Perhaps it got into an ancestor cow's drinking water or wafted through the air to be breathed in by chickens or pigs downwind and became part of those animals' genetic inheritance. It means you just might be taking in toxins with your morning bacon and eggs or your evening crispy chicken. Some experts even recommend removing the skin of fish before eating, especially freshwater fish.

About the only way to ensure absolute and complete protection from the possibility of dioxin exposure from food is with a strictly vegan diet, but of course, as noted, don't eat your vegan meal out of plastic containers.

A number of common objects and articles, implements and gadgets, quotidian utensils and odds and ends may also contain risks. For example, one chemical in the group of nonpersistent pollutants is BPA—bisphenol A, a synthetic chemical compound found in those infamous plastic bottles and food containers, in sports equipment items, and even on the inside of food and beverage cans. Worst of all, there may be BPA in the lining of water pipes in some areas of the country. Water filters, anyone?

On the plus side, there is at least one very easy way to avoid BPA. You know those thermal paper receipts they hand you at stores, restaurants, gas stations? They are actually coated with BPA— one reason, perhaps, that BPA is one of the most widely produced chemicals on earth. That makes it hard to avoid, so when the checkout clerk asks if you would like a receipt, say no, thank you. Iris says no, teaches her kids to say no, thank you, and if the clerk extends the receipt to her anyway, she holds open the bag for the clerk to drop it in. That's what we mean when we say that you have the power to control a great deal of your environment.

And yes, BPA is a known endocrine disruptor that has been shown, in animal studies, to be a factor in autoimmune conditions like endo as well as across a range of health and development problems. So it is good news that, thanks to a 2012 ruling by the Food and Drug Administration, BPA's use in baby bottles is strictly prohibited.

Another family in the persistent pollutant group is PBDEs, or polybrominated diphenyl ethers. Used in flame-retardant products, these compounds show up in building materials, furnishings, electronics, cars, airplanes, textiles, and—again—plastics. They are known to have potential impact on human fertility, so the next time you buy pajamas for your kids, buy the kind *without* the flame retardant.

Then there is triclosan, not to mention its close relative, triclocarban. These "antimicrobial" agents, first used as hospital cleaning scrubs, were soon found in a range of "personal care" products as well as in cutting boards and children's clothing. In 2016, both compounds were banned from use in consumer soaps as potential endocrine disruptors and as resistant to antibiotics. But they still can be found in toothpaste, deodorants, cosmetics, and some cleansers. Stick to hot water and soap, and use a glass cutting board.

Ever hear of phthalates, another group in the nonpersistent family of pollutants? Hard to pronounce, they are nevertheless easy to find—in shower curtains, floor tiles, some medical equipment, building materials (again), children's toys, perfume, makeup, moisturizer, nail polish, liquid soap, and hair spray. Phthalates too are endocrine disruptors—possible metabolic disruptors as well.

Avoid:

BPAs
PBDEs
Triclosan
Triclocarban
Parabens
Phthalates

The list goes on. Small hits to your health, perhaps, but your health is already compromised due to endo. It makes sense to avoid further vulnerability, doesn't it?

Again, we're not trying to scare you. Really. But it's important that you be aware of how downright *normal* a lot of these substances are. Given that there are an estimated seventy thousand synthetic chemicals in commercial use as of this writing and about two thousand more being created each year, it is a tad impractical to memorize every synthetic chemical on earth. The idea is, step by step, to rid your own environment at least—at home, at work, at play—of the things that may be doing you harm. You can replace them with other things. For example, instead of buying yet another brand-name water in a plastic bottle—a bottle that then gets added to the pile of "recyclable" garbage—just buy a "clean" water bottle once and fill it from the tap each time. Iris's pick is Lifefactory, a glass bottle in a protective sleeve so it won't shatter if you drop it, but there are lots of stainless steel and other "green" choices out there.

The point, as is true for just about everything having to do with endo, is that you are not powerless. You control a great deal of your environment, and everything within your control, you can change.

Amy concedes that it was her patients who first nudged her to be mindful of everything in her environment. "What do you clean the bathroom with?" they would demand. "What's in that lubricant you use?" It was a quick and well appreciated lesson in how certain kinds of ingredients can burden an autoimmune condition and exacerbate the inflammation process.

Today, both of Amy's offices are as free of chemical-heavy cleaning products and phony fragrances and potentially harmful materials as they can be. Amy claims that, as of this writing, the offices still have not reached perfection, but she keeps working at it. Ditto with her home, and ditto with the activities and projects she can control—for example, in every situation where her children are concerned.

For Iris, it started with the allergies and eczema her daughter went through as a baby, prompting what would eventually become, over a process of years, a totally organic way of eating and living for the entire family. It was, she says, an evolution, not an overnight revolution. As her kids grew, and as Iris and other young mothers began sharing the alarming data about dangerous "stuff" in their children's environment, keeping those dangers at bay became an all-out, all-inclusive, full-time project the Orbuch clan embraced wholeheartedly.

If our spouses and children can adapt to these changes, so can women with endo. And just as our families are doing better as a result, so will you.

Keep in mind, though, that where both our families are concerned, the changes continue step by step over time.

PERSONAL CARE

It's just as Revlon founder Charles Revson said long, long ago: "In the factory we make cosmetics. In the store we sell hope." Women have been buying it since time immemorial, and we all want it, but when women with endo buy hope in the store, they also need to keep in mind what is being made in the factory.

Why? What's the worry? It's not like we use enormous amounts of these products, and we're not exactly eating them.

Actually, we are. How many times a day do you refresh your lipstick? Is there any way some amount of what you apply to your lips is not entering your mouth and being ingested? Granted, it seems an infinitesimal amount—but for how many years does a woman use lipstick? And did you know that many commercial lipsticks contain lead?

Then there's lotion. Sometimes we slather it on. Sometimes we massage it in "deeply." The slathering and deep massaging could include the phthalates, antimicrobials, and synthetic chemicals we try to avoid in pesticides, in plastics, and certainly in our food. And there is research suggesting that nanomolecules of these kinds of products, smaller than can be seen even microscopically, can somehow seep into the body and enter the bloodstream.

Or we spray on a fragrance, the manufacturer of which is under no legal compulsion to disclose its ingredients and may therefore be combining as many as twenty possibly volatile compounds. Among those compounds, you are likely to find synthetic chemicals derived from petroleum that you then obviously breathe in—and hope that your lungs filter *out*.

These days, there is a new marketing language to meet a rising demand for products that won't be damaging to people or the planet. The industry is meeting the demand with trendy new products advertised as "organic," "natural," "plant-based," or "bio-active."

Beatriz Alegría is a professional journalist (as well as a blogger and editor)* with more than ten years' experience covering the natural beauty scene who says those marketing claims are effectively meaningless. In Europe, the law is far more stringent about what the words on beauty products mean; in the United States, however, "organic," "natural," and the like are advertising slogans without any particular meaning at all. European law also requires that ingredient lists must include every single ingredient, while US law does not. Some three thousand synthetic chemical compounds banned in Europe are allowed in the United States, which means the research and label-reading assignment for the conscientious endo sufferer is a lot heavier and more consequential on this side of the pond.

It also means that endo sufferers in the United States cannot know for sure what personal care products may be doing to them. Nor is there any way to prove that such products may be specifically harmful to women with endo—except that we know that a great many contain endocrine disruptors, which can certainly exacerbate endo symptoms.

In the case of personal care, therefore (which is, not to put too fine a point on it, so *personal*), we offer a simple, sensible recommendation: Make a clean break from the products you've been using that may contain endocrine disruptors and replace them with products known and guaranteed to be clean, natural, and organic—switch to what Beatriz calls "green beauty." She made the

---

* Editor of www.newyorkforbeginners.com.

transition years ago. Like so many consumers, she wanted products created by companies that could demonstrate both an environmental and social conscience along with a commitment to women's health.

Obviously, your transition will be highly individual, as each woman's preferences and practices are about as unique as signatures, not to mention that they change with the seasons, circumstances, and time.

But be aware ahead of time that the transition to green beauty may challenge a lot of ingrained and fairly universal assumptions about what personal care offerings can and should do for you. For example, many popular makeup products use silicones to smooth away wrinkles, so if you give up those products, you may have to accept some lines and creases. By the same token, switching to a "clean" shampoo—that is, one without chemicals like sulfates—may mean saying farewell to that frothy mass of suds your mother told you was what made your hair "squeaky clean." It wasn't. It just made a frothy mass of suds—and very possibly stripped oils from your skin in the process. The bottom line is that you may have to change your expectations about what these products will do for you.

Begin with the product you use most frequently and work your way down the list. Typically, that's a deodorant/antiperspirant; it's something we apply generously, and it routinely contains endocrine-disrupting ingredients. Give yourself permission to sweat a little—maybe start the change in the fall or winter—and be assured that there will be no odor.

For each product that you want to swap out for a natural/green substitute, Beatriz suggests experimenting for at least a month. It takes that long for skin to renew itself completely, and the time gives you a chance to assess how well you like it. Beatriz took a year and a half to throw away everything and create a new beauty routine for herself—a reasonable amount of time.

Start with products certified organic by the U.S. Department of Agriculture, which is responsible for policy, laws, and regulation of agriculture-based products as well as of farms and food. Any product it certifies organic has passed rigorous requirements for both content and methods of production; fully 95 percent of any USDA-certified product is organic, while the other 5 percent meets *very* high standards. That makes USDA organic products a good launchpad for your transition to green beauty—the perfect template on which to build your own stockpile of personal care products.

Beatriz offers another essential bit of advice—namely, "Don't make yourself crazy." Reading the label wrong, failing to understand it, or just giving up on the research happens to us all at one point or another.

Not every green product choice will work for you. Beatriz knows this firsthand: She got hung up on a shampoo boasting sulfates-derived-from-coconut, which sounded great for someone with sensitive skin on her scalp, but these particular sulfates-derived-from-coconut had been highly processed, and the result was something so far from coconut and so irritating to the skin that she ended up throwing away a mostly unused bottle. Everyone's skin is different and responds to skin-care products in its own way.

Is there a faster way of finding the right products for you than a one-at-a-time process of elimination? Sure: Throw out every product currently in your medicine cabinet and order anew from sources that sell only clean personal care products. There are more and more such companies popping up all the time. It is a considerable investment, but if you suffer from endo, it may well be worth it.

The Green Beauty Marketplace

Here are a few retailers of clean beauty products; many have brick-and-mortar stores as well as websites:

www.badgerbalm.com
www.credobeauty.com
www.rmsbeauty.com
www.thedetoxmarket.com
www.paiskincare.us (a London-born, British brand)
www.beautycounter.com

When it comes to specific products, here are some of Beatriz's favorites:

DEODORANTS: Schmidt's has regular baking soda-free options for sensitive armpits. Pachi is another manufacturer I like; they were also the first to come up with an underarm detox mask to help transition from a synthetic deodorant to a natural option.

BODY CARE: Dr. Bronner's castile liquid soap and solid soap bars are among the cleanest options out there. Erbaviva's USDA-organic body oils and Dr. Bronner's organic body lotions are wonderful moisturizers. Pure shea butter works well on dry skin patches.

HAIR CARE: The cleanest option available is to wash your hair with Dr. Bronner's castile soap, but it has to be followed by a thorough cider vinegar rinse to seal the hair shaft. Acure has some really good shampoos that have a minimal amount of safe synthetic ingredients. They also have styling products.

FACIAL SKIN CARE: Finding an effective green skin-care routine takes a lot of trial and error, as the needs of the skin vary depending on external aggressions (the effects of the seasons in terms of heat, humidity, and cold; the levels of pollution; the exposure to blue light coming from computers, and so on); and internal needs (such as your stress levels, the hormonal cycle, the amount of sleep you get, and the medications you are taking). Here are some tried-and-true products I keep on rotation:

- Pai's Avocado and Jojoba Hydrating Day Cream
- Bottega Organica's Elevate Face Oil
- MŪN Akwi Purifying Cleanser
- Rosewater spray to act as a toner
- Badger sunscreen
- RMS Beauty

AT HOME

A friend of Amy's lives in one of those residential high-rise buildings making up the Manhattan skyline. She came home one day to find a notice at the building's entrance announcing that asbestos mitigation was taking place. The building's construction probably dates to a time when asbestos was legal and in common use. If your home is an older construction and asbestos is a concern or suspicion, you can hire experts to perform the appropriate tests; check the Yellow Pages.

Inside the house, the aim should be that the next time something breaks or wears out, you will replace it with a clean version.

In the kitchen, for example, rethink your use of plastic, and aim to replace plastic with glass as much as possible.

In the bathroom, check out the shower curtain and bath mat. What is in these things that you may be breathing in or repeatedly coming into contact with? Next time you shop for these items, find healthy substitutes.

Mattresses in your bedroom can be expensive to replace. But it can't hurt to check those mattress tags we're not supposed to remove "under penalty of law" to see if your mattress might contain flame retardants or PVC or polyurethane foam. You may want to replace it with an organic mattress one day, but meanwhile, there are lots of workarounds to mitigate any harm: mattress covers, pads, barrier cloths, even old sheets.

Throughout your house, are there rugs or carpets? Curtains? Wooden furniture with puffy cushions? When it's time to redecorate, think "green" when you shop for the new stuff. And when it is time to repaint your house or to restain the exterior or to spackle defects in the walls, be aware that there are "green" options in paint and stain products as well. If you can, do it the green way: use non-VOC paints and stains; it means they are free of volatile organic compounds, unstable chemicals that release gases the EPA ranks as harmful to people and the environment. Most of the time, these healthier paints and stains are only a few dollars more per gallon than the harmful kind—a worthwhile expenditure.

Bottom line: We are in no way suggesting that you spend a fortune on an organic mattress or tear apart your entire home from ceiling to floor and start from scratch. Not even close. What we do want is for you to be aware that the home you love might indeed contain substances that just might be affecting your well-being. Start with that awareness, and step by step, think about removing products containing those substances and replacing them with stuff that does the same job but without the potential for harm.

THE HOUSE-PROUD ENDO SUFFERER

Household cleaning products, as you know by now, are also a source of chemicals that can fuel the disease process of endo. So part of cleaning up your environment is making a clean sweep of these supplies as well.

It doesn't hurt to repeat the warning that terms like *organic, non-toxic,* and *natural* mean both anything you want them to mean and therefore nothing at all. A product advertised as *organic,* for example, can sometimes contain a pro-inflammatory substance, while anything *fragrant* tends to require the mixing of a chemical cocktail of unknown ingredients. In essence, it's hard to promise spotlessness without synthetics.

Two excellent sources of overall guidance and product information in this area—vis-à-vis both do-it-yourself cleaning products and truly green commercial products—are the inimitable Environmental Working Group (www.ewg.org) and Women's Voices for the Earth (www.womensvoices.org). Be aware also that many "clean" cleaning products are available in chain stores like Target.

As a general, easy rule, stay away from: formaldehyde, ammonia, chlorine, sodium hydroxide, perchloroethylene, and a group of substances called glycol ethers, which are used as solvents, and which include 2-butoxyethanol (EGBE) and methoxydiglycol (DEGME). If you see any of these on an ingredients list, don't buy the product. Be sure also to avoid household bleach, which releases dioxins—toxic to every endo sufferer—as a by-product.

(You might also want to make your morning coffee using un-bleached paper filters; dioxins are key to the process of bleaching paper products.)

KNOWLEDGE IS POWER:
FINDING WHAT YOU NEED TO KNOW

Products and their distributors will happily note on their websites as well as in retail stores that a product is USDA-certified organic. The creators of that product worked hard to obtain that certification, and they and their distributors know there is a growing, discerning market for products that can boast such certification. It's a major marketing tool.

The USDA Organic Integrity database (http://organic.ams.usda .gov/integrity) is a way to research the agriculture-based operations at the *start* of the process of providing agriculture-based products. That makes it an important source but not exactly one useful for quick and easy tracking of consumer products. Instead, it's a place where you can do research on a specific certified organic farm or business, or search for an operation with specific characteristics. And while the site provides an abundance of information (including a spreadsheet of operations certified in a particular month in a particular year), the database itself is dense and time-consuming to work with.

Both the federal government and state governments typically have departments of health, consumer protection, public safety, agriculture, and environment—if under a range of different titles. And they all have websites—for *almost* every state, type in your state's official abbreviation dot-gov (e.g., tn.gov, ny.gov, ks.gov)—

which can all be helpful in researching standards and who meets them.

There is also an array of nonprofit organizations offering certifications for different kinds of products. Madesafe.org, for example, screens products for toxic ingredients. Savvywomensalliance.org also recommends brands for a safer and healthier home. In all cases, we recommend you check out who is on the board of the organization and who their organizational partners are. If industries being researched are heavily involved, think again.

The champion of them all, to be sure, and the organization we recommend wholeheartedly and without reservation is, as noted, the Environmental Working Group (EWG), at www.ewg.org. Its guide to the Dirty Dozen Endocrine Disruptors is a must-have for any woman diagnosed with or suspected of having endo. Print it out and carry it with you at all times. Equally valuable are the EWG's Shopper's Guide to Pesticides in Produce and rankings of some two thousand household products, along with quick tips and an essential label decoder for choosing healthy, environmentally safe and sound products. It's really the place to find everything you need or want to know.

Above all, be sure to download the EWG's set of mobile apps—in particular, Healthy Living. You can scan a product's barcode or input the name of the product to see EWG's take on it. For a personal care product, it will tell you the ingredients; assess the level of allergy concern, cancer concern, and developmental concern; and provide an overall score in which the higher the number, the higher the hazard. Food scores consider nutrition, ingredient, and processing concerns, then create an overall score—1 is high, 10 is low.

Feel confident that you have the tools to build a clean, safe environment for yourself and your family, as well as to feed them clean, safe food. Those are two of the most important weapons to get you locked and loaded against endo. Among other benefits, that confidence can help calm your stress and cool the jets of your up-regulated central nervous system—a case of adjusting your *external* environment to help soothe your *internal* environment, an essential element in getting yourself well ahead of your disease.

ENDO AND YOUR
STATE OF MIND

The power of the mind to influence physical health has long been known, one way or another, but now hard science is defining the connection in depth, shedding new light on our understanding of wellness, and helping forge new strategies for achieving it. For endo sufferers, the implications are profound.

The core of the hard science, as we learned back in chapter 7, is that pain happens in the mind through the processing of information about a message of danger coming from somewhere in the body, with the brain eventually "deciding" whether or not the danger warrants a response. This processing relies on some mechanisms that can inhibit a response and others that can activate a response, and the result can go either way. Actually, it can go both ways, which is why pain sometimes fades in intensity or goes away altogether: The injury or insult that stimulated the danger message hasn't changed; the processing of the message has changed.

Over time, as we also know, pain responses can sensitize the central nervous system, impairing the mechanisms that inhibit the pain response and energizing the mechanisms that activate it. Eventually, as sensitization keeps on extending and amplifying the pain response, it causes an actual change in the connectivity of the neurons, and, as Dr. Sheldon Jordan explained, the pain response effectively becomes chronic.

In short, the brain has a lot to answer for when it comes to the pain that afflicts our bodies, souls, and lives. So it's fair to ask: Can the brain disarm its own pain activation mechanisms and build up its pain inhibitor mechanisms?

Modern science says yes, affirming what Aristotle guessed and Freud explained, what virtually all faiths promise and self-help books offer: techniques and practices to modulate your state of mind, shifting the connectivity of neurons back the way they were before or reconfiguring them in a new way. The modulating action is called neuroplasticity—in other words, the ability of your brain to change throughout your life.

There can be a negative effect to all this, as we and all healthcare providers know because we see it all the time: A patient comes in with a fairly straightforward physical disorder but has a history of anxiety, depression, obsessive-compulsive disorder, or all three, and what should have been a simple cure becomes anything but. Simply put, a physical disease is made more challenging if the patient has a mental or emotional disorder on top of it—feeling blue makes the headache feel even worse multiplied many times.

But neuroplasticity can also help you deal with your disease. Where endo is concerned, it means your brain can literally help lessen the pain in your pelvis and desensitize your central nervous system. Of course, it cannot cure your endometriosis. But, along with exercising therapeutically, making better choices about your nutrition, and managing what is manageable in your environment, these techniques and practices may indeed help you live more comfortably, productively, and—dare we say—happily.

The forms that mindfulness techniques and practices can take run the gamut—from the ancient Greek philosophers' search for ataraxia (absolute calmness) to modern-day Zen, from navel-gazing to table tennis, from sitting alone in the quiet of your room to solo-climbing El Capitan—with ropes, please. A great many of the techniques and practices are or derive from quite ancient methodologies and beliefs of Eastern cultures, especially of India (yoga) and China (qigong and tai chi). These practices, basically spiritual in nature, reflect a penchant for autonomous self-fulfillment, achieved through a high level of mental focus on inner stillness or calm.

What does mindfulness ideally achieve? The standard answer is: being present in the moment. What that means is of course open to interpretation, but certainly it means that if you are in a canoe on a lazy river on a beautiful day, you do *not* turn your mind to all the stuff you failed to get done yesterday and will need to finish up when you go back to work on Monday. Instead, being present in the moment in the canoe on the river means that are you taking in the sights and sounds around you; you are directing your attention to where you are and what you're doing. In other words, you are concentrating on now. As the saying goes, depression lives in your past—failure to get the work done yesterday—and anxiety in your future—what you face on Monday. Today, in the canoe, just paddle and focus.

But of course, that's easier said than done, particularly if you're in pain. The brain's natural tendency is to multitask. All that time sitting in a canoe offers the brain ample opportunity to fixate not only on what you left undone in the office but on depressing past pain you have suffered, and to anticipate with anxiety not only what's ahead on Monday but also whether the pain you feel will ever truly end. Juggling the two balls of past pain and likely future pain—while also keeping you aware of where you're paddling right now—uses up a lot of processing effort. But if you can dismiss the past and future and focus solely on the present, the brain calms down. Handling just the one ball—the present paddling—is not nearly as taxing as juggling three; it doesn't use as much processing power. On the contrary: It is both soothing and restorative. It can be healing. The only catch is that you must make yourself do it.

Casie Danenhauer, doctor of physical therapy, registered yoga instructor, and a retreat leader who often works with those suffering pelvic pain, says that being and feeling present is consistent with a steady intention: to create space. Space between past and future; space between the mind wandering and being fixed on a single focus; space between breaths, between thoughts, space that is even just a moment of stillness in the heart. It is in that space that the state of being present happens—sometimes not when you're striving to capture it, but when you simply allow yourself to receive it.

Iris attended one of Danenhauer's pelvic health retreats as an "outside" observer, propelled there thanks to a patient she had treated for endo. The patient had come to Iris with just about every co-condition the disease can produce; she was also depressed and anxious. Yet she committed herself to our multimodal program, following it to the letter, and she managed to fully regain her life within an astounding six months. When Iris asked what had been the turning point that had propelled her to commit herself to this healing, she answered instantly that it was Casie Danenhauer's retreat. Iris was intrigued; if it worked for one patient, why wouldn't it work for others? She decided to attend one to see how retreats might add perspective to her practice.

Casie introduced her to the other participants as a neutral, remote observer and asked that they all respect Iris's dispassionate, research-based presence. But it didn't take long for the communal practices to draw Iris in, and the power of these exercises over time proved revelatory. The dispassionate researcher was feeling more grounded, more rested, and, ironically, more productive and more available to the people she cared about—from her patients to her family and friends—than ever before. Iris felt almost literally transformed, and she returned home from the retreat with a new understanding of what constituted "enough" and a new power to cease striving/moving/racing, to become present in the moment, and to achieve all she sought to achieve far more joyfully.

You don't necessarily need a three-day retreat in the desert to learn to be present in the moment—although it couldn't hurt. In fact, precisely because anyone can learn this kind of mindfulness—with practice—it has become a key instrument in the science of pain management. It is a way to start peeling back the physiological changes that central nervous system sensitization has wrought—the restrictions on pain inhibitor mechanisms, the up-activation of pain responders—and begin restoring healthy neuronal connectivity.

There's another essential point worth making here: Because for many women, physical pain—not to mention medical treatment or maltreatment—creates trauma, the validation of psychological damage through mindfulness or therapy can validate the physical pain as well, and this can open channels of communication between patient and doctor. Anger at being in pain worsens the pain and impedes healing. It is why both of us very often refer patients to pain psychologists or recommend retreats—Amy actually has run retreats for dealing with pelvic pain—as well as "prescribing" mindfulness practices.

HOW

Dr. Alexandra Milspaw, a licensed professional counselor and sex-ologist specializing in chronic pain issues—and the co-director, with Amy, of a series of those retreats*—explains how mindful-ness operates as a mechanism of pain management. It is, she says, "the only cognitive exercise that heals and restores the hardware in the brain that actually manages pain." The hardware comprises the parts of the brain that interpret nociception and cause pain perception—that is, the mechanisms for activating the pain per-ception and the mechanisms for curbing it. Milspaw equates prac-ticing mindfulness to "brain physical therapy"; it repairs those pain management mechanisms in the brain the way PT can restore tight muscles to working order. Click the SAVE button on the repair and you start to reverse the pain perception.

The concept is evolving rapidly. A study run by Fadel Zeidan, PhD, of Wake Forest School of Medicine in September 2018, brought together seventy-six individuals, none of whom had ever meditated or done any other kind of mindfulness exercise before. All were measured for "dispositional" mindfulness—a determina-tion of the baseline mindfulness levels that were natural to them. The study participants then underwent functional magnetic resonance imaging (fMRI), during which they received heat stimulation at

---

* Dr. Milspaw and Amy for some years headed a team that designed and operated retreats aimed at helping patients deal with chronic pelvic pain and empowering them for self-care.

120 degrees Fahrenheit—pretty painful, which of course was the idea.

The scans showed that participants who had scored higher on dispositional mindfulness levels experienced less pain. The researchers' analysis of this ability to not get "caught up" in the experience was that the "higher dispositional mindfulness . . . was associated with greater deactivation of the posterior cingulate cortex—which plays a prominent role in pain and episodic memory retrieval."[19] (Episodic memory retrieval is mind-wandering, as opposed to cognitive activity.) If this deactivation of a key player in the brain's pain perception mechanisms is the case with brains that are mindful by disposition, it raises a fairly obvious correlative question: Can you train the brain to that deactivation of the posterior cingulate cortex—with some sort of mindfulness exercise—and get similar pain perception results? Could increasing mindfulness through training provide relief of chronic pain?

A number of studies already suggests it can. First, says Alex Milspaw, there is research showing that training the brain definitely makes a difference; Milspaw cites studies noting physiological changes in the brain "within ten to fourteen days of practicing mindfulness for twenty to thirty minutes a day." So that's the first step: you can train the brain, through practice, to be more mindful.

Another study may be telling us *how* that happens. Reported in 2016,[20] this study likewise involved participants who had no prior mindfulness experience—twenty-six of them. They were assigned to practice a twenty-minute audiotaped guided exercise in mindful attention to the breath (MATB) every day for two weeks. The practice is simplicity itself: Sit quietly someplace, maybe close your eyes, and just breathe normally but with focused attention on your breathing. Attend mindfully to each breath, to what it feels like as your chest rises and falls or as the air moves in and out of your nose or mouth. Breathe in, breathe out. If your attention wanders to a sound or a thought or your to-do list, gently bring it back to your breathing. Don't expect anything, don't force anything, just allow it to be. Breathe in, breathe out, and when you're ready, open your eyes.

After two weeks of this training, the participants underwent fMRI scanning while being shown distressing images. In some cases, they were asked to practice the mindful-attention breathing while they watched; at other times, they were instructed to view the images passively.

Again, the functional scans showed significantly less negative effect when the participants practiced the mindful-attention breathing. Specifically, doing MATB while looking at negative images appeared to decrease activation of part of the amygdala but increase the connectivity between the amygdala and the prefrontal cortex. It calmed the amygdala and opened a highway from the calmed-down amygdala to the prefrontal cortex.

The amygdala is the part of the brain that processes emotions like fear, anxiety, and aggression. The prefrontal cortex is more of a mystery, but most neuroscientists suspect that it has something to do with executive function or cognitive control. What the MATB study showed researchers was that this double-whammy effect of mindfulness training—i.e., both deactivating the amygdala and up-activating its "integration" with the prefrontal cortex—constituted "a potential neural pathway of emotion regulation."[21]

The bottom line is that mindfulness training works to modulate pain and ease the state of mind pain may precipitate. You can affect your state of mind to affect your state of health—at least, the state of how you feel.

Big disclaimer here on our parts: We are not brain experts in any scientific sense. In fact, the brain remains fairly uncharted territory in the world of science, although it's a frontier that, as these studies demonstrate, is being extended every day and in many diverse ways. But these research reports, along with many similar studies, are easily translated: They suggest very strongly that mindfulness practices, in their range and variety, can lessen pain perception, cooling parts of the brain associated with pain and opening new pathways for pain diminution. In the most human sense, in the realm of healing in which we both operate, this means that your state of mind really can affect both your pain and your state of well-being—your health. That makes mindfulness an essential discipline in the multimodal program we believe can help beat endo. It doesn't cost a penny, requires no special equipment, and you can do it on your own whenever and wherever you choose. All that's needed is your commitment.

MINDFULNESS TRAINING

There are many different kinds of mindfulness practice—so many that you are bound to find at least one that suits you—meaning one you will do on a regular basis because it works with both your lifestyle and the particular state of mind you are prone to. We are in no way recommending one over another; rather, we want to explore how a range of different practices, when combined with therapeutic exercise, good nutritional choices, and a safe and clean environment, can help alleviate your pain, cool your central nervous system, and strengthen your power to beat your endometriosis.

Alex Milspaw, for example, speaks about and teaches both passive and active mindfulness practices. In both types, you're engaged as the agent of the practice. In an active mindfulness practice, you may be more physically or energetically involved, but as with a passive practice, you are inside the practice without judging it.

Table tennis—Ping-Pong—is one example of an active mindfulness practice. It requires your total focus on batting back that tiny ball; there is little room left in the brain for anything else. Swimming also counts as active mindfulness. The focus is on breathing and on counting your breathing.

Another active mindfulness suggestion is a self-operated game of "I Spy" using all your senses. Simply catalogue in your brain everything you're aware of in this moment, expressing silently but in language what you see, hear, smell, taste, and touch.

Try it right now.

Instant "I Spy"

Answer these questions:

What do you see as you read this page of this book?
What can you hear right now?
Breathe in and say out loud what you smell.
What can you taste?
You're holding this book or reading device; what is the feel of it?

Creative effort has always demanded absolute focus, making it an ideal path to active mindfulness, so by all means activate your artistic yearnings and make a painting, throw a pot, compose or play music. Reading a book counts too.

Where some of the more athletic forms of mindfulness practice are at issue—the solo climb of El Cap would be one example—we add an important caveat: If you have any musculoskeletal issues—hip or back dysfunction, joint dysfunction, or the like—proceed with caution and under the guidance of your physical therapist, or maybe just chill when it comes to physically active mindfulness and do the passive form till the issue has been dealt with. You shouldn't just "power through" your pain; listen to your body.

Meditation—that is, the act of attending to one focal point for one portion of time—is at the heart of passive mindfulness. Meditation is simple, can be done anywhere at any time, and requires only your brain and body and carving out time and space dedicated solely to the process.

Get Ready to Meditate

Find a spot where you can be comfortable and still.

Turn off the phone—or at least put it in airplane mode.

Turn off your answering machine, your stove timer, your tablet, television, radio—anything that pings, anything that might sidetrack you or divert your attention.

Focus your mind on slowing down your mind. Or focus on your breath. Or on a picture in your head of a place you love. Nothing else.

Stay present—in that space Casie Danenhauer described. Don't wander into the past or the future.

The brain calms, and you feel a stillness that is refreshing.

Yet doing meditation is often not as simple as it sounds. A good way to begin is with guided meditation; a number of terrific apps available for free can help you start such a practice. The voices guiding these apps may ask you to visualize a scene or offer gentle instructions for entering a meditative frame of mind. Keep at it, and over time, you'll learn to recite the guidance yourself or will have found your own way.

In fact, the internet has become a bit of a gold mine for mindfulness seekers. Here's a partial list of meditation guidance apps:

Headspace

Calm

Breethe

iRest

Lumosity

Recognise

Buddhify

Certainly, there is an argument to be made that active and passive practices are two sides of a single coin. Yoga would seem to embrace both. Its linking of breath to movement—passive to active—is what makes it so powerful, yet it seems to dismiss the distinction between the two forms in its search for balance.

Two other ancient Eastern practices also prize balance (physical, emotional, and spiritual): qigong, which is active physical movement like tai chi and yoga, and acupuncture, which is passive. Both these practices are aimed at balancing the flow of the life force within you, and both, but especially acupuncture, are regularly applied for pain management and stress management.

Qigong, a practice going back more than four thousand years

and sometimes referred to as "moving meditation," combines highly stylized fluid movement with slow, deep breathing and often with chanting as well. The movement is always intentional, breathing is rhythmic, and calm prevails, as you aim to achieve mental focus by visualizing the qi—your life energy—moving through the pathways of your body, guided by your mind.

As for acupuncture, while it cannot be said to treat the disease of endo, it is one of the ways a woman with endo can calm her central nervous system and thereby advance her healing process.

Perhaps the best known of the ancient Eastern practices, at least in modern-day America, is tai chi—full name, *tai chi chuan*. If you have ever been to China—or to New York's Central Park on a weekend morning—you are likely to have seen tai chi in action. The slow, graceful action of movements accompanied by deep breathing is very often performed by quite elderly practitioners, for it is comfortable at any age. It can be a truly beautiful sight to watch these tai chi practitioners, alone or in a group, as they focus their minds on the conjoined flow of their breathing and their motion. They do not stop moving; they do not pause. It is all one flow of movement: arms, legs, core, mind. Originally a self-defense practice—a very ancient martial art—tai chi puts minimal stress on joints and muscles and lowers the stress level in your mind and body as well. It demands and teaches muscle control, balance, a steady blood flow, and being absolutely present in the moment.

Whatever mindfulness practice you choose, and whether you are confronting pelvic pain or a bad day at the office, tightened abdominal muscles or a relationship going sour, these practices can still the flurry or fill the hollowness within. They're a key weapon in beating endo.

Amy's Mindfulness Practices Picks

Yoga

A hike, bike ride, brisk walk, etc.

Positive self-talk and distracting yourself—with a card game, dinner with your BFFs, a museum visit, etc.—whatever gets you outside of your pain

Any pain-free sport: tennis, skiing, snowboarding

Iris's Mindfulness Practices Picks

Yoga

Ocean swimming

Kickboxing

Walking the dog

Sitting in an infrared sauna listening to Pandora's Meditation Spa Radio

Shabbat: From sundown every Friday to sundown every Saturday in celebration of the Jewish Sabbath, Iris unplugs from computers and phones, puts aside the frenzied compulsion of the week, and recharges, returning to her connection with family, friends, and her religion

YOGA AS THERAPY

If the ancient yogis who created the practices and forms of yoga thousands of years ago could come back and see the multiple modifications that Westernization has brought to their spiritual practice, they probably would shake their heads in disbelief—and possibly in dismay. Hot Yoga, Power Yoga, Standup Paddleboard Yoga, Yoga for Weight Loss, Yoga for Bad People: The variations seem endless. In a number of cases, they also seem a long way from the "definition" of yoga in a text from the first millennium BCE: "the stillness of the senses, the concentration of the mind, . . . creation and dissolution."[22] Yet yoga is perhaps the most popular of all the mindfulness practices today, its power consisting in the way it links breath to movement, passive to active.

Casie recalls that her first connection with yoga was as a gymnast eager to "get my exercise on" and strengthen and enhance her already trained muscles. She has gone well beyond that focus now, but yoga-as-physical-fitness remains a common starting point for many people.

But it is yoga as a therapeutic tool that is our focus—the yoga of that ancient definition, the yoga that is pretty much the exemplar of the mind-body connection. It's all about that bidirectional "communication" up and down along neural pathways. We both do yoga, Iris regularly and Amy intermittently, and when we do, we both feel we are retreading the tires of our minds, quieting our bodies, and restoring a kind of ardor to spirits that sometimes sag with fatigue. If that's not therapeutic, what is? But of course, what we are talking about is the kind of therapy that provides not just restoration but also prevention, not just rehabilitation but also pain management—everything for a patient to get better, whatever can make a patient well.

Dr. Ginger Garner first started using yoga back in the 1990s in both her physical therapy and athletic training practices and believes that yoga is the "missing piece" of today's approach to pain management. This doctor of PT, certified and licensed athletic trainer, mother of three, and community activist also founded the world's first yoga-inspired interdisciplinary training program for licensed healthcare professionals, the Professional Yoga Therapy Institute, and is the author of *Medical Therapeutic Yoga*. Approaching yoga as a scientist, not a guru, helps her explain what it can do for pain management.

Simply put, yoga's particular role is its power to affect the vagus nerve. The vagus is the longest cranial nerve in the body and, as its name implies, it wanders all over the place. It links the brain stem to the heart, lungs, and gut; it interacts with key organs; and it controls a huge number of conscious and unconscious body functions. You cannot taste or weep or do much of anything else without the vagus nerve getting involved.

Specifically, says Garner, there are five mechanisms of pain that yoga can alleviate via the vagus nerve: inflammation, the sympathetic nervous system, oxidative stress, brain activity, and opioid receptors. You can imagine how wide-ranging the impacts of this might be. Just think what the implications might be for adding yoga's deep breathing techniques to the weapons fighting our current opioid crisis. The yoga breathing "treatment" would influence the body's opioid receptors naturally, which, Garner points out, "is cheap, it's low-tech, it's safe, it's easily administered, and it can influence activity in the cortex with no side effects."

That makes yoga a potentially formidable addition to the fight to beat endometriosis because, unfortunately, opioids are routinely prescribed for women with undiagnosed endo—particularly during those well-known seven to twelve or so years of misdiagnosis—by doctors who see no alternative and do not realize the long-term impact. Such treatment can literally alter the brain's response to pain, making that pain even more oppressive and far more difficult to treat properly, as our colleague, neurologist/pain specialist Dr. Sheldon Jordan, explains: "Patients treated with opioid medications such as oxycodone and hydrocodone will often develop a paradoxical worsening of local pelvic pain or a total body pain syndrome." Jordan says, "They have sleep disturbance, mood changes, severe exercise intolerance, and profound sensitivity to even light touch." Bowel and bladder complaints "may also be worsened."

The need then is to get these women to free themselves of the opioids—itself a difficult, painful process, but essential before just about all other treatments for endo and its co-conditions—certainly surgical intervention—can be applied. All those treatments are perforce put on hold "until the patients are entirely off of opioids," according to Jordan.

Certainly, yoga breathing would be a far better first approach to the pain of endo—to any pain—than these opioids.

We cannot urge it strongly enough: Take yoga's power and send it into battle against pelvic and abdominal pain and all the many co-conditions of endometriosis. Pair it with the potency of physical therapy. Add it to the rest of our protocol of lifestyle changes in nutrition and in what you surround yourself with in your environment and in proper treatment of the disease. Because of how it can affect the vagus nerve to have an impact on inflammation and the sympathetic nervous system, pit your yoga practice against a couple of heavy-duty targets—one, inflammation itself, the basic condition of endo, and two, the chronic perception of pain that the sympathetic nervous system carries.

In fact, says Garner, yoga's influence on vagal nerve activity is inversely proportional to inflammation; the more we influence the vagus nerve through yoga, the less we experience inflammation. Where the constant perception of pain is concerned, yoga's influence on the vagus nerve can actually reverse the perception by combating the blood vessel constriction and muscle tension that chronic pain induces. All this plus its ability to influence the opioid receptors without pharmacological compounds make yoga's influence on vagal nerve activity incredibly valuable.

One caution, however, is that yoga postures on their own will not exact the full range of emotional, behavioral, and hormonal changes needed to induce vagal modulation. Instead, Garner suggests adding one of two modalities—or both—to ignite that modulation: breathing and sound, both known for their impact on vagal nerve activity. If sound as an igniter of pain modulation seems odd, think about someone grieving or in pain, as Garner suggests; chances are the person has assumed a rocking position, may be moaning, may be sighing—stress relief responses, all of them. "Paced humming or sighing layered over paced breathing" not only produces the effect that stimulates vagal modulation; because of the way it works mechanically, it can also directly affect the pelvic floor in particular, releasing any tension there, making it an important tool in pain management and pain relief for pelvic health. For Garner, breathing and sound are the essential ingredients to let yoga "really work" its power to affect the vagal nerve and, as part of Garner's interdisciplinary approach, can bring on the relaxation response and undo the stress of endo pain.

TALK TO YOURSELF—POSITIVELY

There is one more mindfulness practice we want to bring to your attention: positive self-talk, buttressed by intentional positive distraction. Among the other attractions of this simple practice, it is convenient, absolutely free, and you don't have to leave home to do it. All you have to do is talk to yourself—in your head, not out loud (although out loud works too)—which we frequently do anyway; in this case, though, we must think ahead and bring a positive attitude to the conversation.

Amy is particularly interested in this mindfulness technique because of the nearly 250 patients her practice treats per week. Their physical gains can be slow and hard-won, which often goes hand in hand with negative attitudes and high anxiety. Positive self-talk can help.

For example, there are those patients who somehow convince themselves, typically after a single session, that the physical therapy isn't helping. They leap from that to the idea that nothing can help and that they are doomed to live in pain forever. That becomes a pattern, as a single negative reaction gets reinforced through negative self-talk (not that years of pain could be "cured" in one session of PT or of anything else!). The reason is simple: When you talk to yourself, there's no one there to contradict or stop you. You can catastrophize endlessly, and the negativity will continue to spiral downward, taking you and your pain and your ability to counter the pain with it.

Talking to yourself positively can begin to reverse that negative thought process. Amy has seen it work in her practice, and she knows it can be seen in the fMRI scans of people in pain. The light in the brain that turns on when a person is in pain literally dims when the person tries positive self-talk. *Yes, I'm in pain, but I have a plan for alleviating the pain* can go a long way toward, in fact, alleviating the pain.

A good way to bolster the effect of positive self-talk is through distraction—forced distraction if necessary. By that we mean making yourself sit down to watch television—preferably something mindlessly entertaining. Or taking yourself to a movie, or to a museum or gallery, or to the zoo—anything that takes you out of yourself and away from your pain. Then make that part of your positive self-talk: *I watched two hours of* The Good Place *and enjoyed it so much I totally forgot I was in pain, so clearly, that means that I* can *feel pain-free, and it also means that I* will *feel pain-free again . . .*

It is another example of the brain's power over how we feel. By reminding your brain of the constructive and optimistic actions you can effect on your own behalf, positive self-talk is another mindfulness practice that can literally affect your health for the better.

EASY DOES IT

Whatever mindfulness practice you choose, remember not to practice it too hard. You don't want your attempts to relax to stress you out further. Remember Amy's response to emptying her brain for what she hoped would be a nice meditation session? Her to-do list poured right back in with a vengeance; attractive as meditation seemed, it never quite worked for her. Over time, it was invariably a hike in the woods that put her brain at ease. Iris too recalls that it took a lot of yoga practice for her to find her ease. In mindfulness as in most things, patience can be a virtue.

There is no more powerful organ in your body than the brain. It can absorb, capture, learn, synthesize, interpret anything and everything that can be perceived. Emily Dickinson said it perfectly:

The brain is wider than the sky,
For, put them side by side,
The one the other will include
With ease, and you beside.

Mindfulness practice helps you keep the brain wide, and that is the state of mind you want regulating the state of your health.

EXCISION SURGERY

None of the lifestyle changes we've talked about—nutrition, environment, mindfulness—change the fact of your endo. It's still there.

None of the treatments you may be trying make the endo go away either. Not birth control pills, not Lupron, not norethindrone acetate, not an IUD, not Orilissa (the most recent contender from Big Pharma). As Iris explains, all these treatments are suppressive rather than curative; that is, they simply manage symptoms. Meds just do not treat endo—period! In fact, Lupron and Orilissa put you in a menopausal state and may have long-lasting and unpleasant side effects. So if controlling symptoms is the aim, stick to Iris's go-to recommendations: birth control pills—either the 24/4 type or continuous doses—or the Mirena IUD, which goes directly into the uterus and releases a steady state of progesterone right where it can do the most good.

But again, any relief from symptoms does not achieve the eradication of your endometriosis. In fact, the disease may still progress even while you are treating its symptoms. So when patients on medical treatments tell us that "my endo got fixed, but now it's back again," we need to correct them. No. That's not what happened. What happened is that some form of treatment lessened the symptoms temporarily, but the endo was still there. Even the work of physical therapy—absolutely essential for pain management and for overall musculoskeletal health—doesn't rid you of endometriosis.

What does actually eradicate the endo in your body is surgical excision—that is, cutting it out of you. That surgery is the cornerstone of beating endo. All of the physical therapy and lifestyle changes this book asks of you are necessary in order to prime your body so as to ensure that surgery's greatest success. As we've noted before, Iris won't perform excision surgery—her specialty—unless and until the patient's central nervous system is sufficiently cooled and her muscles are sufficiently lengthened—in other words, unless and until her body has gotten to the point where surgery can best succeed. *After* surgery, everything that you did to prime your body must be continued—the physical therapy plus making the right choices in your nutrition, environment, and mindfulness practices—in order to make up for how the disease affected you over however many years it was in your body. You won't fully beat endo without maintaining the practices that keep the co-conditions at bay.

Yes, there are two surgical procedures available for doctors to recommend: ablation or excision. As you well know by now, we emphatically and unreservedly advise the latter.

True, one of us is an excision surgeon, a specialist in the procedure who has performed it on women of varied ages and at different phases of their illness and would naturally advocate its use. But the other of us is not a surgeon; rather, she is a physical therapist who has worked with pre- and post-op patients of both procedures and has noted the profound differences between them. Amy's ablation veterans tell her that their pain subsided briefly, then came back with a vengeance or, just as often, moved to another part of their body. Either way, the pain cycle kicked in again, sensitizing surrounding muscle, tissue, and organs—the whole central nervous system.

After excision surgery, however, when patients follow Iris's prescription to go back to PT post-op, both Amy and the patient can sense how much more effective the therapy is; over time, minimal therapy achieves maximal results because the underlying cause of the viscero-somatic pain reflex is gone, the anatomical distortion has been righted, and the reflex is becalmed.

EXCISION IS NOTHING LIKE ABLATION

The two procedures are fundamentally and almost startlingly different. They are not equal in the nature of the procedure or results. In fact, we don't think the two can be equated in any way, shape, or fashion.

First, let's look at what the two procedures are about. The word *ablation* comes from a Latin verb meaning to take away; *excision* comes from a verb meaning to cut out thoroughly. Ablation does the taking away of endo by cauterizing or burning off the surface of the implants. Surface is all it takes away. It's a superficial procedure. Excision, by contrast, cuts as deep as needed to remove all the endo. Both procedures are minimally invasive and performed laparoscopically—that is, using a tiny camera inserted into the navel. In ablation, an instrument hooked up to electricity then burns off the surface of the lesion. In excision, the surgeon removes the implants from the root, cutting away—Iris's instrument of choice for the procedure is scissors—until only healthy tissue remains.

It's estimated that 95 percent or more of surgical procedures on endo patients are ablations. They are quick and easy; no specialist training is needed, so just about any primary care obstetrician/gynecologist can perform it. A prolific doctor can do as many as eight ablations a day.

Back when Iris was a young ob-gyn doing her residency, the ablation procedure was not only the "norm," it was practically the sole surgical procedure performed for suspected endometriosis. Following her residency, Iris moved on to her fellowship with Drs. Reich and Liu to focus on honing her skills in excision surgery. This was in-depth specialist training, which requires both volume and consistency. Its aim is to create a particular skill set and expertise—very different from the equally essential skills and expertise of a generalist. Where a generalist has a wide range of knowledge—how to deliver a baby, perform a C-section, treat hot flashes, what to do about a breast lump—the very breadth of knowledge required means that the generalist cannot delve into the depths of expertise in which a specialist must be at home. In the time Iris spent mastering her precise specialist skills of excision surgery, she also witnessed firsthand the outcomes of those surgeries, and there was no question in her mind: Excision patients did far better than did those who had undergone ablation. Simply put, excision patients were positioned to get well; ablation patients weren't.

In the meantime, however, Iris was preparing, post-fellowship, to conduct her first grand rounds. As part of the process, she combed the literature for pertinent data and came upon a study comparing ablation and excision. The study looked at what were described as women with "stage 1 and stage 2" endo and more or less affirmed that ablation and excision were equivalent. The study, entitled "A randomized trial of excision versus ablation for mild endometriosis,"[23] was performed in the United Kingdom by a fellow of the Royal College of Obstetricians and Gynaecologists,* the UK's premier professional association for ob-gyn practice. The research concluded that there were "no statistically significant differences between the two procedures"—no appreciable difference in outcome at all, except that ablation could leave behind more cell damage.

Iris was stunned by the results, which flew in the face of what she herself had observed, but she was even more profoundly stunned by the methodology: The paper had looked at only twenty-four patients—hardly a sufficient number to count as a representative sample. In her scientist's mind, the n—the number of people sampled in a study—was insufficient for drawing a proper conclusion— a conclusion, as it happened, totally opposed to what her own eyes had shown her.

At the time, however, the study accorded perfectly with what both doctors and patients wanted—fast and facile pain relief—and confirmed ablation's status as the norm when it came to the "next step" in medical intervention on endo patients. Fast forward to the present and finally to prospective, randomized, double-blind data showing that excision "provides symptom reduction for up to five years,"[24] while a review article concluded that twelve months after surgery, "symptoms of dysmenorrhea (painful periods), dyschezia

---

* Jeremy Wright, who authored the study, has before and since its publication made enormous contributions to the field of endometriosis and minimally invasive surgery.

(painful bowel movements), and chronic pelvic pain secondary to endometriosis showed a significantly greater improvement with laparoscopic excision compared with ablation."[25]

Yet despite that, even now, ablation remains the pervasive choice recommended and carried out by the majority of ob-gyn and primary care physicians—that is, doctors educated as generalists and trained to manage their patients' diseases. To Iris, it makes no sense that despite good science proving that excision works better, women with endo continue to suffer through wrong treatment and the wrong surgery. What does make sense is empowering women to take charge of their health. That is what impelled her to write this book.

SHALLOW VERSUS DEEP

The difference—that ablation literally skims the surface while excision just as literally cuts deep—is essential to understanding the advantage of excision.

Ablation burns off only the tip of the iceberg, so to say; the bulk of the endo implant is still there, undisturbed beneath the burned-off surface. Most of the generalists and ob-gyns who perform the procedure identify targets for ablation based on the scant information about endometriosis they received in their medical school textbook—namely, to look for implants with "a chocolate-brown color." That is not sufficient for finding all the endo, as was made vivid in Amy's story way back in chapter 1 about the International Pelvic Pain Society meeting in Sydney in 2005, when almost everyone in the audience failed to recognize the many colors of endo.

In fact, the ablation procedure acts almost as an engine of recurrent surgeries. It's why doctors like Iris hear so many veterans of ablation complain that their endo has "come back." As we noted earlier, it hasn't come back; it never went away in the first place. It simply wasn't treated properly. Undoubtedly, it was not correctly identified, and therefore a bunch of endo was left behind. Iris recalls one patient who had gone through nineteen ablation procedures, each providing mild relief for a brief period of time. For that patient, the first ablation procedure opened a pathway to multiple surgeries that only ended with Iris's successful excision of her endo, thereby establishing a "clean slate" on which the patient could build herself back to health.

That clean slate is the result of the excision specialist reaching widely and cutting deep. The specialist surgeon searches everywhere in the peritoneal cavity and has been trained to spot implants reflecting a rainbow of different colors and appearances—blue, red, white, yellow, clear—and to cut and remove them all, leaving behind only healthy tissue. The generalist, remember, rarely looks past the "chocolate-brown" he or she learned about years ago.

As with just about any surgical procedure, both ablation and excision cause scarring—although far less in excision. The sticky adhesions of the scar tissue formed in ablation can create their own problems in time, tugging at the peritoneal "covering," further distorting the pelvic anatomy, which in turn distorts the pelvic floor and the abdominal muscles even further. (This is when you want the kind of mobilization techniques Amy and her staff can perform, releasing the tightened muscles and "unsticking" the stuck-together tissue.)

The bottom line of these aftereffects—i.e., the implants continuing to grow and new scarring occurring—is that ablation simply does not work as a healing measure. In the absence of a cure for endometriosis, it's still not a solution an endo sufferer can count on. Its alleviation of symptoms is likely to be temporary at best, and its benefit to a patient's overall health is brief and minimal—if that—and in fact, given the potential for scarring and further anatomical distortion, its effect is adverse.

For both of us, it's difficult to square the inadequacies of the ablation procedure with the frequency with which it is performed on endo patients. We understand that no one wants to undergo surgery. It's a trauma to the body, there is always a risk, it requires anesthesia, and there will be pain in recovery—which will take time to diminish. But there is no doubt in our minds that if and when far-reaching medical attention is warranted and wanted, it should be excision surgery—accompanied of course by steady attention to all the lifestyle disciplines we have written this book to advocate.

"ONE SURGERY DONE RIGHT"

One surgery done right—Iris's motto—is neither particularly quick nor easy. It's not the sort of procedure a surgeon can perform or a patient undergo in the time between when either of them drops her kid at his piano lesson and picks him up when it's over.

Equally essential to the scheduling, of course, is the surgeon's assessment that the patient's central nervous system has been sufficiently downregulated. "Desensitization has to precede surgery," as Dr. Sheldon Jordan has said, and only when Iris herself has judged that the de-escalation has proceeded far enough to ensure a successful procedure will she go forward. Operating too soon, as Jordan has noted, could mean cutting into tissue not yet suffi-ciently "cooled," which might conceivably exacerbate a still fraught condition.

Similarly, during the course of the procedure, there can be no rush. Iris doesn't wear a watch in the operating room. While there is no imaging modality to gauge how much endo she may find and therefore how long the procedure might last, her physical exam and review of records will have given her some idea of what awaits. But the surgery will take as long as it will take—"Not a minute more," as Iris tells her patients, "and not a minute less." Similarly, you can never be certain how much time the surgeon's own preparations will take, or how long the consultations with the OR nurse, anes-thesiologist, and pathologists will last, or when the various pre-op rituals will wind down.

Iris begins on her feet at the patient's bedside, typically holding her hand as she asks her to "tell me about a happy place; describe it," as the anesthesia is initiated. Patients constantly tell Iris how much they appreciate this personal touch and being guided to "go under" by happy thoughts. But in truth, there is an important medical benefit to stressing the mind-body connection right there in the OR at the moment of surgery. In addition to studies that confirm this, Iris's own observations are clear that making this connection before the patient goes under means far less pain med-ication needed once she comes out of it.

Once the anesthesia takes hold, the patient has to be properly positioned on the table—Iris pads the patient's nerves and limbs so they are not under undue stress—and then a catheter is inserted to keep the bladder decompressed, as well as a uterine manipulator so she can move the uterus, get to the endo, and restore normal anatomy. She then makes a small incision in the navel and inserts the camera. From there, its lens can pan across the entire peritoneal cavity, and the images show up on television screens placed strategically around the OR. Iris then makes a few other small incisions—about five millimeters long—and through a hollow sleeve called a trocar inserts a grasper, scissors, and a cautery tool in case it's needed. If the procedure is being done robotically, she docks the robot and sits down at a console that allows her to take hold of a gizmo not unlike the joysticks she mastered as a video gamer in her teens, and, focusing through the viewfinder on the console, will begin to survey everything the camera can see in three-dimensional high definition. Rest assured: Iris is doing the surgery, not the robot, and she's using advanced instrumentation, which actually has wrists that bend and 3-D visualization—instrumentation far superior to that of traditional laparoscopy.

Whereas many doctors put the scope straight into the pelvis and start searching the ovaries right away, Iris prefers to follow a kind of pilot's checklist of all the organs and coverings to be viewed. She looks everywhere, from the domes of the diaphragm to the liver, gall bladder, appendix, all of the small intestine, large intestine, and all of the pelvis—everywhere. It's a sort of survey of the anatomy—with an eye out for any distortions of that anatomy that might indicate the presence of endometriosis or any other causes of pelvic pain. She finishes by looking inside the bladder; she leaves no stone unturned.

After that overall survey, Iris zeroes in to identify the endo she will excise, guided by her expertise and experience in the signs and signals that can indicate the disease.

The first hint is an increased blood supply. Because endo implants must be "fed" by blood if they are to grow, increased vascularity, as it is called—that is, an excess of blood vessels—is a clue to the presence of implants.

She'll check the uterosacral ligaments; does one or the other appear thickened or asymmetric? Such thickening can be an indication that endo has infiltrated the ligaments—another hint of a good place to start excising.

Certainly, brown lesions on the ovaries are a classic sign of endo, the standard indication of its presence that "all doctors recognize," says Iris—generalists and specialists alike. But she looks well beyond that textbook description to explore for blue, yellow, black, white, and red lesions. White endo lesions she knows to be older; they have a thickly scarred fibrous appearance, as if they have been around for a while. Black and red lesions are newer.

She'll also look for what is called an Allen-Masters Window, a puckering in the normally smooth, shiny, cellophane-like covering of the peritoneum. The puckered look is a signal that there is probably endo in those folds and wrinkles.

Of course, she will zero in on any scarring as an indicator of endo that has been around a while—or perhaps of a past ablation procedure.

And she will look very carefully for clear vesicles—that is, small, raised, lesions. This colorless evidence, as we shall see in chapter 12, is essentially what endo often looks like in teenagers, and it is all too easy to miss. One of the great advantages of robotic technology is precisely that the 3-D, high-definition camera, as opposed to the 2-D laparoscopic camera, enables a stunningly high degree of visual power and precision.

Whatever Iris identifies she excises robotically with the scissors, operating this instrument with a level of precision and thoroughness unachievable otherwise. The images in 3-D and high-def provide her a better, clearer view than her own eyes could secure—it is almost like being inside the patient—while at the same time control of the scissors enables almost perfect

exactitude. There is even a tremor filter in case the surgeon's hand
grows tired and starts shaking—although Iris has never experienced one.

Endometriomas—that is, cysts within the ovary that are filled
with endo—are a common finding in women with endo. Generalists performing surgery on endometriomas use a pop-and-drain
technique that ends by burning the cyst wall, actually killing a
good number of eggs and adversely affecting fertility. It also sets
the patient up for later surgeries—even months later in some
cases—because the cyst was not fully removed.

Iris, however, meticulously separates the cyst out from the normal ovary and removes it in its entirety. It's a favorite procedure for
her because the technique she applies uses hydrodissection—high-
pressure water instead of cautery—to separate the normal ovary
from the cyst, thus minimizing damage to the patient's eggs.

Finally, when all of the excising is done and all specimens
have been sent to pathology—results will take another seven to
ten days—the patient heads for the recovery room and, barring
complications, in most cases goes home that day. Of course,
every individual is different post-surgery, but Iris advises patients
to take it easy for a week—no work or school. She also advises
patients to restart physical therapy after that first week of rest to
help the pelvic floor muscles. No vaginal or rectal PT work for
four to six weeks, of course, but it's important to begin to ease the
cramped-up, clamped-down muscles of the pelvic floor as well as
of the abdomen, thighs, back, diaphragm, and any other affected
areas from head to toe.

Even once patients are back at work, Iris suggests they take it
easy for four to six weeks in order to let those tiny incisions heal
and to lower the risk of hernia. Patients are exhausted post-surgery;

they have gone into surgery on an empty tank, and the procedure has further taxed their bodies. It's why Iris tells her patients to "listen to your body." The body heals from within, and if it tells you to flop down on the sofa and sleep, do so: Pay attention to what it tells you so it can heal. But as we both advise, simply moving around is encouraged. Just don't overdo it.

It is also true that for women who have had multiple surgeries and/or who suffer from multiple co-conditions, healing and recovery take longer than for others. Everybody is different.

It's equally important to make sure the patient's surgeon and her physical therapist are in sync on how to progress. In fact, it typically takes a team to treat endo; Iris, for one, thinks of herself as a quarterback and is in regular communication with her patient's PT, urologist, pain psychologist, gastroenterologist, pain management doctor—whoever is on the team.

As for the excised endo, it's gone. It won't "come back" in that same spot. This is one reason excision has been called "the gold standard" for surgical treatment of endometriosis. It is why Nancy Petersen calls it "step one" in addressing endo—step one of the many steps needed. And it's why it is the backbone of our multimodal approach. That program must continue as an inherent part of your life after surgery. Sixty percent of healing takes place during the first six postoperative weeks; full healing is complete at three months. Those three months are critical, so it is important to adhere 100 percent to all the other disciplines that you carried out before the surgery and that we've written about throughout this book: physical therapy, nutrition, environment, mindfulness. Continue it all.

Accompanied by those disciplines, excision is, to date, the single surgical procedure that can be a key tool in beating endo.

Surgery for Adenomyosis?

Excision surgery performed on a woman who may have adenomyosis as well as endo will treat only her endo; she may still be left with adenomyosis symptoms. If so, and if the woman still wants to ensure future fertility, we offer two potential methodologies to alleviate her symptoms.

One is our multimodal program. Iris has found that adenomyosis responds well to the wide-ranging lifestyle changes we have detailed in these pages. It means that the woman who follows the program may sufficiently cool her central nervous system that, following excision surgery, her adenomyosis will be the sole pain generator left in her body. Our hope is that the discomfort of that pain would be relatively manageable until she sorts out her childbearing plans.

The other possible methodology is a progesterone-releasing intrauterine device (IUD), "officially" used of course for contraception but a great option for medical management. We recommend it with one caution: Just as with endo patients, women with adenomyosis often have tight pelvic floor muscles, so we counsel that physical therapy, for however many sessions it may take to relax the pertinent muscles, is essential before insertion.

Both research and our personal knowledge confirm that the progesterone-releasing IUD can be extremely effective for controlling the pain of adenomyosis till the woman is ready to have her children.

A SPECIAL CASE

Endo and Teens (but This Chapter Is Not *Just* for Teens!)

Earlier, we introduced you to our "typical patient"—a woman who most likely has suffered debilitatingly painful periods since middle school, went on to develop painful bladder and GI problems, "graduated" to pelvic floor and other musculoskeletal dysfunctions, and by now is also suffering from depression, anxiety, and the whole palette of endo disasters.

What if we had "caught" her back when she was first having those cramps at age thirteen or fourteen? What if, before her pelvic muscles grew tight with pain, before she came to accept constipation as something normal, before her mother dragged her to the third or was it fourth different specialist in as many months—what if, before all that, she had come to practitioners like us? The difference in the health and well-being she could be experiencing right now would be enormous. The difference in the future she could look forward to would be seismic.

How seismic? Researchers are just beginning to scope out the breadth of lives that would be retrieved, rejuvenated, and set on a path to health if endometriosis were diagnosed early, as a spate of recent studies has made clear. "Laparoscopically confirmed endometriosis is found in 70 percent of girls with painful periods," a 2015 study revealed,[26] and a 2017 study claimed that "adolescents are *more likely than adults* [our italics] to present with non-cyclic pelvic pain."[27] They also, prevalently, present with nausea. So teenage endo is not simple. Indeed, a third study, also from 2015, found that "both early and advanced forms, including deep endometriosis, have been reported to be present in teenagers."[28] And the study goes on to suggest that deep endometriosis may have "its roots in teenage years."

The conclusion from these studies and the lesson they teach could not be more straightforward. Early diagnosis is critical. And to expedite care, so is "timely referral to a gynecologist experienced with laparoscopic diagnosis and treatment of endometriosis."[29] For parents, pediatricians, school nurses, teachers, guidance counselors, and anyone else in touch with teenagers, if you come up against a girl presenting with or complaining of really bad menstrual cramps, think endo. She is likely—70 percent likely, as the research makes clear—to have the disease. The time to act is right now.

This is precisely why we find it so gratifying to treat young patients. It is why Iris believes that her main goal as a gynecologist is to find endo early and save these girls from years of misdiagnosis and its accompanying suffering. It is why both of us see early diagnosis as our chance to help young girls stem the damage of endo before they have suffered too much for too long—and to put them on the path to the healthy, fulfilling lives they deserve. Getting to them early means that their musculoskeletal structure has not yet become totally clenched and their neuromuscular system still has "bounce" and flexibility. The central nervous system has only begun to upregulate, or it may not yet have even started to dial up. The bladder and bowel might still be working more or less okay. Chronicity has not yet set in, so there is a good chance to reverse course.

Moreover, lifestyle behaviors that may affect the girls' overall health adversely are not yet totally entrenched or ingrained; teenage minds and bodies are still supple enough to learn the sustainable behaviors that can support health and well-being over a lifetime.

All of this makes this time of life an appropriate juncture at which to undertake any interventions that can make a long-term difference in the quality of these girls' lives.

Both of us have recently seen an increase in patients of this age group—although they rarely come to us via a pediatrician's referral. It's as if some sort of standard, clichéd thinking kicks in that says gynecologists are for women, physical therapy is for athletic grown-ups, and pediatricians focused on vaccinations, childhood diseases, and injuries need not be attuned to signs and signals of a disease that is commonly associated with "bad periods" and infertility.

Fortunately, these patients find other paths to our offices.

The way it usually happens is that a parent, typically the mother—often a mother who herself suffered severe menstrual cramps as a young girl—becomes alarmed that her young daughter is undergoing such severe monthly pain and is missing so much school. Mom makes an appointment with the pediatrician, who prescribes some form of birth control—pills, most likely. These pills impede the natural rhythms or fluctuations of the female hormonal flow, instead creating a hormonal steady state. When hormones are not cycling, the pain of menstrual cramps may diminish. The teenager's periods may be less painful, and if her periods have been heavy, they can lighten.

Yes, she may suffer side effects: her blood pressure may rise, and she may become even moodier or more confrontational—enough to reject the whole idea of the pills. But basically, the pills can manage her symptoms—that is, so long as she complies properly with the protocols for their use. Not easy. Birth control pills are either monophasic, each pill containing the same measured dosage, or triphasic, with graduated dosages each week for three weeks, and they come in 21/7 packs, which means you take the pill for twenty-one days, then have seven days off, or in 24/4 packs, twenty-four days of pills and four days off. Pills are Iris's go-to prescription for alleviating symptoms—along with a reminder that they do not cure endo and, in fact, that even if symptoms improve, the endo is still progressing. The prescription she typically gives is for a trial period of about three months, and if all goes well, for continuous pills after that. But birth control pills must be taken at the same time each day, and adhering to a rigid schedule isn't always easy, convenient, or realistic for young girls with a plate full of academic, extracurricular, and social demands.

The reality, as we all know, is that even the most responsible teenagers sometimes forget or just blow off being compliant with complicated things like pill protocols, just as they don't always make their bed each day or walk the dog as they swore they would. It means that compliance tends to fall by the wayside, to yield to sleeping in late on a weekend morning or forgetting to bring your pills with you for the Saturday night sleepover. Result? The teenager's hormone level dips, and the uterine lining is shed from the uterus, causing spotting and bleeding, possibly painfully.

This is one reason that Iris suggests that her young patients take the pills at dinnertime, when they are *usually* at home or in any event awake and upright, and that they set the alarm function on their phones to ping every minute for ten minutes at the stated time—*and* to use the "most obnoxious-sounding alarm" as the alarm ping. Anything that helps—because the truth is that if these girls don't take the pills properly and on time, the pills just won't work.

After a while, the mother of a sketchily compliant teenage girl probably decides it's time to take her daughter to her own gynecologist, but there's not much help there either. Maybe the doctor switches the twenty-one-day/seven-day on-off pill package to a twenty-four-day/four-day on-off schedule, which is better in general for endo patients, but that of course does not fundamentally treat endometriosis; it continues to manage symptoms—that's all.

Then Mom begins to take in that her daughter is complaining of "stomach problems" and seems to be going to the bathroom way too often. Come to think of it, this has been the situation since the girl was about eight, well before menstruation. Seeing no connection between her daughter's GI issues and her awful menstrual cramps—why would she?—the mom takes the girl first to a gastrointestinal specialist, then to a urology specialist. Drink more water, these doctors say. Eat more fiber. Worst case, give her MiraLAX; they sell a special dosage for kids.

It goes on, until finally, the moment comes when the frustrated and probably exhausted mother says to herself, *What on earth is going on here?* and she invokes the twenty-first century's great guru and ultimate sage—Dr. Google. In other words, she searches the internet for information about painful and heavy periods in adolescents, and somewhere among the recipes and sponsored ads and Facebook posts, she sees the word *endometriosis* and decides to consult a gynecologist who specializes in that condition, whatever it is—even if it means traveling thousands of miles.

That is typically how teenage girls come to see endo specialists like Iris.

It is safe to say that both the girls and their mothers are stunned that just about the first question Iris asks is about any history of constipation or bladder issues before the painful periods began. They may also wonder why, after palpating the teenager's abdomen, Dr. Orbuch remarks on "super-tight muscles." What does any of this have to do with menstrual cramps forcing a teenage girl to miss a day of school once a month?

A GROWN-UP DISEASE IN AN ADOLESCENT

We titled this chapter "A Special Case," then proclaimed in the subtitle that it was not just for teens. We are neither hedging our bets nor trying to have it both ways at once. Endo in teens is a special case for two reasons: One reason is that, as a culture, we still don't like talking about these kinds of "female" topics at all, but especially where youngsters are concerned. The other reason is that despite the recent upsurge in teenage patients in our practices, they still represent a tiny portion of diagnosed endo sufferers and so constitute a special case by reason of size.

But the fact is that we all can learn a lot about the disease of endometriosis by looking hard at its occurrence in teenagers, and that is why this chapter is not just for or about these girls; it is about endo and how it advances and where it might have begun.

Back in chapter 1, we referred to a study of fetal autopsies indicating that 9 percent of female fetuses had endometriosis. That percentage rings a bell because an estimated 10 percent of fully mature women—actually, anywhere from 10 percent to 12 percent—also have the disease; as we have noted frequently, the rule of thumb is that worldwide, almost one in ten of us has endo.

One possible cause of the endo in these female fetuses, as the study's authors suggested, was that the mothers might have been exposed during their pregnancy to some form of dioxin or similar endocrine disruptor—proven causes of endo. But another powerful conclusion was that the mother or grandmother or great-grandmother or possibly a male ancestor of one of these afflicted fetuses genetically transmitted the endometriosis. We know, for example, that a teenage girl whose mother or grandmother or aunt had endo has a sevenfold to tenfold higher likelihood of having the disease herself than do her peers.

But whatever the teenage patient's genealogy, by the time her mother has brought her to Iris's office, her profile looks something like this: She is sixteen, her period began when she was eleven, and the cramps have been persistently awful ever since. But of course, menstruation is not the start of puberty, just a key part of it. In fact, estrogen levels have been steadily rising in the young girl's body over several years, causing gradual change—breast buds, underarm hair, pubic hair. More than likely, other estrogen-driven developments also took place but did not show up on the surface of the body, which is why when Iris asks about any history of stomach issues, she is not surprised that the answer is "Yes, stomachaches and constipation since she was eight or so." Nor is she surprised at the tightened abdominal and pelvic muscles; she figures the girl's abdomen and pelvic floor are already dysfunctional as she probably has been straining on the toilet as well as clenching forward in the fetal position against the pain of her stomachaches for a couple of years at least. Further examination, if okayed by both mother and daughter, equips her to pinpoint the girl's endo as in the area between the rectum and the vagina, and she surmises that inflammation there is the source of the girl's intestinal woes and rectal pain. An exam is not necessary, however; a patient's history alone and the intensity of her menstrual pain are typically enough for a doctor like Iris to suspect the presence of endo in these teens and adolescents.

But until Iris, no one—not the school nurse who pretty much dismissed the girl as a hypochondriac, not the pediatrician, not the gynecologist, not the urologist or gastroenterologist, not the pediatric shrink the mom thought might help—no one has connected the dots of the different symptoms or thought they had anything to do with one another. So for this mother at least and for the patient as well, receiving an actual diagnosis, hearing a name attached to the girl's suffering, offers relief.

PARENTS AND THE "ENDO WHAT?" QUESTION

The first task of parents whose young daughter has been diagnosed with endo is education: what the disease is and can do, why it is accompanied by co-conditions, which co-conditions their daughter already has, and yes, fertility may be an issue in the future.

With younger teenagers in particular, it's important to discuss with mother and daughter whether a vaginal examination is necessary—that is, if it is going to add to what can be gleaned from asking questions. Certainly, a lot of information can be gained through an abdominal exam and a thorough conversation. Moreover, girls who use tampons may well be comfortable being examined internally, although the exam on girls of this age tends to proceed more slowly and far more gently than with mature women, and it includes careful explanations every step of the way. For Iris, the mother of two daughters, this age group is her "niche"; they are a population she "has always loved," and she finds it easy to connect with teenage patients—and with their parents.

Still, there is no way that learning that your daughter has endometriosis is an easy lesson for mothers and fathers to absorb. No parent wants to think of his or her child suffering in any way, and in the case of a teenager with endo, her mother may also assume a burden of guilt.

The truth is that there is not a lot of hard data out there about adolescent endometriosis. Our friend and colleague, the pioneering Mary Lou Ballweg, oversaw a 2003 study that found that endo symptoms were starting earlier than was generally thought— before the age of fifteen. That was a hint that the starting age for menstruation was going down, and the study also projected that symptoms would become increasingly severe as that starting age continued to drop.[30] Not exactly what a parent wants to hear. So it is important to assure parents of the good news—namely, that their conscientious attention to their daughter means that the disease has been "caught" early, in good time to stop or slow deleterious effects and in very good time to develop a treatment plan that can give the young girl her best shot at a fulfilling, healthy life.

Obviously, it is equally essential to educate the teenager herself. These girls need to understand that their endometriosis continues to progress despite all the potential symptom alleviation they are getting through birth control pills, physical therapy, and the lifestyle changes that Iris will also prescribe. They need to understand our multimodal approach and that its benefits will only be maintained as long as they stick to it. They need to understand further that their well-being, right now and in the future, is within their control.

In other words, a teenager with endo must do just what we have recommended for mature women with endo—the full program that is the core of this book.

TEENAGER PT

Physical therapy for young teens is a lot like physical therapy for adults.* What is particularly satisfying about treating teens is that the interventions are typically easier and the results come much faster than with adult women. That's because these bodies haven't yet become "so adaptive to the guarding reflex, the incorrect postures, the bad toilet habits," says Amy; "they simply haven't had the time."

The therapists who work with these young women know that even one more year without PT would make it harder to retrieve musculoskeletal health, so they are actually ensuring that the girls stave off some of the worst of the muscle tightness that is par for the course in adult patients. The therapists also know they are helping prevent the shortened abdominal and pelvic floor muscles that would characterize these girls in five more years of inattention, even in one more year. They feel they are stalling and maybe even stopping the chronic impacts of the disease and its subsequent co-conditions. That is a good feeling for physical therapists—inspirational.

---

* For teenagers who are not sexually active, internal manual therapy is rarely recommended; if it is deemed to be essential, both guardian and patient must consent to and be comfortable with its use.

At the same time, says Amy, the PT sessions are opportunities to educate these girls about all they can do for themselves—both in instructing them on how to relax the pelvic floor muscles to help with pain and with bladder and bowel functions and in showing them PT exercises they can do at home—not to mention offering lessons about nutrition, their environment, and mindfulness. Showing them the extent to which they can take control of their disease helps them maintain a positive attitude. And because results come quickly, a kind of inherent positive reinforcement to all that they're taking on is more or less built in.

PT is also of course essential for pre-op preparation and post-op recovery to optimize the surgical outcome, which brings us to the topic of excision surgery among the teenage cohort of endo patients.

PEDIATRIC EXCISION SURGERY

"Pediatric" is defined as age seventeen and younger, and pediatric surgery takes place routinely in the medical profession for all sorts of reasons on kids of all ages.

In the case of endo, at a minimum, the girl should have done sufficient physical therapy to loosen the tightened muscles *and* should have followed the rest of our program: our recommended dietary and behavioral changes, including mindfulness, along with whatever medical interventions an endo specialist has recommended.

But of course, just about everybody hesitates a bit when surgery is recommended for a young person. Certainly, that is true of parents when it is recommended for their child. Some atavistic fear kicks in, or their pediatrician and sometimes a mother's gynecologist will repeat the myth that no female should have surgery until she has had babies or is ready to have babies. It is past time to send that myth back to whichever medieval century it came from.

The truth is that excision surgery on a young girl is the same as excision surgery on a grown woman—with the very significant exception that the surgeon must know how to look for the clear vesicles that signal the presence of "young" microscopic endo to be excised. Certainly, red and black and white lesions may also be found in these girls, but knowing both how to identify and how to excise the uniquely clear vesicles of the young patient is essential. On the other hand, teens may have the more visible advanced-stage endo as well.

For Iris, what sets these surgeries on teenagers apart is also what makes them so particularly gratifying. It boils down to one fundamental fact: Of all her patients, these young girls do best—in terms of the procedure itself and of the outcomes they experience. This is partly because the disease process of endo hasn't yet distorted their anatomy to the extent that it does in older women. Nor has it revved up their central nervous system. Partly also, it's because of the work the girls themselves do ahead of surgery—work that can be an education in how they will need to proceed after surgery and probably for the rest of their lives. By the time the surgery is scheduled, they have seen the difference that physical therapy can make, and they may even have an inkling that eating pizza and drinking a Coke after school every day is not going to help the way they feel. From the surgeon's point of view, however, despite the adolescent lapses, these are patients whose central nervous systems have been flared only a bit, whose musculoskeletal structure got "fixed" in ten sessions of PT, who, despite the illness Iris is about to cut out of them, have young bodies, and what she is about to do is going to make an enormous difference to their lives. It is typically the first surgery these girls have ever had, so for the surgeon, it means a clean slate; as Iris puts it, she does not have to "clean up other surgeons' ablation procedures."

For those of us who help ready them for the procedure and see them through it, what's so very gratifying is knowing that we are helping thwart endo—halting a damaging disease before it can do worse than it has already done. It pretty much ensures that these girls get the shot at growing and developing they deserve to get.

THE FOLLOW-UP

The surgery does not fix the painful bladder syndrome the girl may have. It does not treat her tight muscles. It also doesn't replace post-op physical therapy sessions for her, nor does it mean she doesn't have to have a future discussion with her doctor about fertility, as the next chapter makes clear.

As with grown women, removing the endo does not on its own address the co-conditions that may have caused pain or impairment. The great danger is that these girls are at a time of life when it can be all too easy to put off, or feel constrained by, or just drop the behaviors that can keep them healthy. It is a time of life when you want and are expected to do stupid things. Doing stupid things is essential to growing into maturity—so long as the stupid things you do are harmless. For girls with endo, the afternoon snacking during high school—the daily caffè mocha at Starbucks, for example—the alcohol-soaked weekend parties in college, and other "normal" rites of passage can be harmful if they become habitual.

But if these teenagers have gotten the message about the co-conditions of their endo and the lifelong need for a multimodal approach to the disease, then it is likely that they will recognize a returning pain, be able to identify which co-condition has stirred it, and get busy again on whatever lifestyle behavior they have allowed to slacken. If they do so persistently, they will have escaped the worst of this disease, and it is our hope that they will live healthy lives that will be as full and rich as they can make them.

ENDO AND
INFERTILITY

For many women, the overwhelming concern raised by an endometriosis diagnosis is infertility. For those women, no other concern comes close—not the pain from the disease, not the limitations it is likely to impose, not the changes they will almost certainly have to make in their behavior and the way they live. It doesn't matter if you're married, partnered, or resolutely single, ready to have kids or far from even considering it. Virtually the first thing a woman receiving an endo diagnosis wants to know, almost as a reflex reaction, is if she will be able to have a baby.

One reason she asks is that the words *endometriosis* and *infertility* traditionally have been inextricably linked. Even today, if you google *endometriosis*, the search results will be sprinkled with the word *infertility*. As clinicians and mothers, we understand the primacy of this concern for our patients and for our readers.

The truth is that yes, endometriosis *may* affect fertility. Conversely, it may not affect it at all. As we have seen repeatedly, every woman's body is unique, and different women experience endo's symptoms in different ways and at various levels of intensity. And of course, there are women with endo who suffer no symptoms whatsoever.

But it is also the case that 40 percent of what the medical profession calls "unexplained" infertility is due to endo. "Unexplained" means that doctors have not been able to find an identifiable cause for the infertility. The sperm are healthy and in motion, the fallopian tubes are open, and there is reason to suspect good ovarian reserve. All too often, this is where the search for an explanation stops—and many times, endo may well be the cause of the infertility. Unexplained infertility, therefore, seems a partial analysis at best, a cursory one at worst. Iris refers to this phenomenon as the "endo hidden in plain sight."

But unexplained infertility becomes explained infertility if the right questions are asked. Those questions, which would concern issues like menstrual pain, heavy menstrual flow, any bowel or bladder issues, painful sex, and the like, provide answers that might suggest the presence of endo.

But not all doctors—certainly not enough doctors, not even enough fertility doctors—are attuned to the possibility of endo as contributing to infertility when they offer options for treatment. One distinguished fertility expert who is definitely attuned, however, is Dr. Kelly Baek, an ob-gyn who was fellowship-trained in Reproductive Endocrinology and Infertility at the Weill Cornell Medical Center's Center for Reproductive Medicine in New York, but who is now based in her native California. Baek's way of assessing a patient concerned with fertility is instructive, because if she sees anything at all that is "off" in the tests she performs and the examination she carries out, she wants to know why. As she puts it, "it's not 'normal' to need IVF; there has to be a reason." Finding the reason—and following every clue to do so—is essential.

If her hands-on examination finds thickened uterosacral ligaments, that's a clue the woman might have endo. If her ovarian reserve is low, is it from a genetic factor—and if not, what is the cause? If the uterus is deviated to one side or the other, is it because of pelvic surgery or from scarring from endometriosis? Are the fallopian tubes patent or dilated? Baek herself reviews the images to check and double-check.

A finding of endo as a contributing factor doesn't necessarily mean Baek won't recommend in vitro fertilization (IVF), but it might. Her aim is "to help someone conceive with the least amount of intervention." To realize that goal, asking the right questions and following every lead are both required. If your reproductive endocrinologist doesn't do that, or if you feel like you're being passed along an assembly line in a one-size-fits-all factory, find another doctor.

TWO EFFECTS

There are two ways endo may affect fertility. One is by its inflammatory power, which creates an inhospitable environment for fertilization of the egg and, if fertilization does occur, for implantation in the uterine lining, as we'll explain further in just a moment. The other way that endo may affect fertility is structurally, through the scarring and adhesions that can distort a woman's anatomy and potentially block the fallopian tubes.

To understand what inflammation can do, let's first review the pathway of normal fertility: The sperm, introduced during sexual intercourse or insemination, ascends from the vagina up through the cervix into the uterus and then branches out to the two fallopian tubes, which extend from either side of the top of the uterus.

If the woman is ovulating at the time of intercourse, an egg is re-leased from the ovaries, and the finger-like projections on the ends of the fallopian tubes—known as fimbria—catch it and channel it into the tubes, where it encounters the sperm. Everything is set: The egg is available, the sperm are there; they can meet, travel to the endometrium, and implant there what will develop as an embryo.

Inflammation can adversely affect just about every step of that process, and as we know, if there is endometriosis anywhere in the vicinity, it can set off a cascade of inflammatory responses. It may simply prevent the egg from getting to the fallopian tube in the first place, essentially killing off the egg, or it may prevent the sperm from getting to the egg. It may, when egg and sperm meet and implant into the endometrium, create an environment that is simply not conducive to implantation. Such an environment is filled with message-signaling cells called cytokines, whose actions we don't fully understand but which can be toxic—certainly toxic to implantation and to every other stage of fertility. It is one reason why many women with endo who do become pregnant miscarry—sometimes repeatedly. In some women, the process gets as far as conception, but the cytokine-filled environment dooms implan-tation.

Endo can also block or disrupt pregnancy by structural means. Scarring on the outside of the fallopian tubes, for example, dam-ages the fimbria, and damaged fimbria can't catch the egg released from the ovaries at ovulation. No egg in the tubes equals nothing for sperm to meet. In addition, endo's scarring, adhesions, and dis-tortions of the anatomy may render sex so painful that the regular sexual intercourse that tends to make fertility likely simply doesn't happen.

In any event, as you can plainly see, there are compelling explanations for "unexplained infertility."

COUNTERMEASURES

Can our multimodal program to beat endo affect or possibly reverse the infertility that endo may cause? We know that excision surgery improves the chances for fertility; it literally cuts out the inflammatory cells that may be impeding fertility and thus lets nature do its thing—i.e., put egg and sperm together. The research is clear on that, and Iris, for one, can point to a long roster of patients who have "failed" at IVF, yet have spontaneously become pregnant after they underwent excision surgery—in many cases, within three months of the operation, usually within the first six to nine months. This is especially the case when the surgical procedure is understood as the central principle of the multimodal protocol Iris insists on to cool the central nervous system and strengthen the body before surgery.

There is also medical research[31] showing that acupuncture, one of our go-to strategies for stress management, can likewise boost a woman's chances of fertility. The stress reduction is part of it, but acupuncture has also been shown to increase blood flow to the reproductive organs and help balance the endocrine system—further encouragement to the chances for pregnancy.

Certainly, where painful sex is a cause of infertility, PT's role can be significant. If the pain has a musculoskeletal origin, or if the issue is pain with penetration, suggesting involvement of pelvic floor muscles or connective tissues, physical therapy can be an effective treatment, as research has shown, for lengthening tightened, contracted muscles or tissue or for dealing with adhesions or scarring that may be impeding penetration. And obviously, making sex possible is a first step toward making fertilization possible.

Beyond that, contends Amy, it is also the case that patients diagnosed with endo and unable to become pregnant have gotten pregnant after physical therapy, although she affirms that any connection "is speculative," and, as she adds, there is no physical therapy protocol for infertility. What she believes physical therapy can do, although there is as yet no research to prove it, is work to release connective tissue restrictions or muscle tightness that may be impeding blood flow to reproductive organs. Impeded blood flow can stagnate the whole reproductive system; the blood just sits there, so the inflammation accumulates, bacteria may build up, and the environment becomes congested very nearly to the point of gridlock. That is *not* an environment conducive to an egg and sperm getting together so that the latter might fertilize the former.

It takes highly specialized expertise and great skill to break that gridlock; Corey Hazama, for one, possesses both* and has succeeded in mobilizing the organs of the reproductive system in a number of patients. In an optimally functioning reproductive system, as Hazama reminds us, the ovaries are moving, the fimbriae of the fallopian tubes wave freely, the tubes themselves are "bellowing" in and out, creating a kinetic chain of contractions and relaxations that move the egg in the right direction. Fascial restrictions and adhesions can disrupt this kinetic chain, and while physical therapy cannot undo the restrictions and adhesions, it can in some cases mobilize the tissue of the organs, which may get

---

* Doctor of Physical Therapy, certified Orthopedic Clinical Specialist, certified Functional Manual Therapist, Pelvic Rehabilitation Practitioner.

things moving again. It isn't a "cure," but it may well help create an environment that boosts fertility.

So, of course, does everything else we have advocated in this book. The right nutrition, an environment free of products or influences that may be deleterious to your health, a mindfulness practice that calms your central nervous system, and of course proper treatment of endometriosis all affect your chances for conception. That is basic, and it should be coordinated with any fertility treatment that your doctor recommends. All of these actions together constitute your best shot for optimizing the environment in which a fetus can be implanted and can grow.

INVESTING IN THE EGG BANK

Call it a workaround, call it a backup plan—but egg freezing is a strategy Iris recommends when she is counseling her younger patients about ways to improve their chances of getting pregnant. They've had the excision surgery; they are endo-free and feeling better; this may be the time, she suggests, to explore the idea of banking their eggs while they are still young and healthy.

Whether you have a partner or spouse or lover or none of the above, it is an idea worthy of serious consideration. Kelly Baek says a number of concerns should be weighed—the woman's ovarian reserve and whether the level of reserve is appropriate for her age, her personal preference for when she wants to have children—for example, whether right now or five years from now—among other considerations. Baek says she "feels strongly" that "women with suspected or confirmed endometriosis . . . should freeze eggs or embryos when they are in their twenties and early thirties to keep their fertility options open."

Be aware, however, that the process of retrieving the eggs from your body is no small undertaking; it can be uncomfortable and time-consuming. And even with some insurance coverage, the cost is high, starting with the egg retrieval process and including monthly or yearly storage fees. So when considering the idea of banking your eggs, you will have to look upon it as an investment—but one that may be very much worth considering.

As with any investment—actually, more than with most—this one requires in-depth research. Iris notes that many IVF centers nationwide offer free monthly seminars in which fertility specialists help you educate yourself about the process. Or, make an appointment at one of these centers for an individual consultation. Remember that you are born with all the eggs you will ever have, and that preserving them is one way to help ensure that you can create the family you want. But find out all you can, then decide if it's right for you. If it is, sooner-rather-than-later is probably good advice.

RECLAIM YOUR LIFE

You know your starting point, and you know the route to follow: Identify, in concert with your endo specialist, every coexisting condition of the disease; create a treatment plan for each; execute the plans until each pain generator has been disarmed, until your musculoskeletal system has been restored to strength and balance, and until your central nervous system has sufficiently cooled for excision surgery if needed. Once you have followed this route, you will be better equipped in body, mind, and spirit to recapture and restore whatever this disease has taken from you. That is our commitment to you.

In return, we ask a commitment *from* you—namely: Give it time. Your endo didn't progress this far overnight, and it won't be beaten overnight either. Improvement, when it comes, arrives in increments—sometimes very small increments. Your progress is not going to look like anyone else's progress, so track your own progress, preferably on a monthly versus a daily or weekly basis, and resist the temptation to compare yourself to others. Beating endo is not a contest; it is a journey.

Iris always makes a point of taking down word-for-word answers when she asks all those many questions at a first appointment: How many times a day do you urinate? How frequently do you have a bowel movement? Is sex painful? One reason is so that, at any stage along the way, pre- and post-surgery, if a patient swears she is following the program yet fears she is not making progress, Iris can ask the questions again and compare the answers: *Six months ago, you were urinating eighteen times a day; now it's down to twelve. You said you moved your bowels maybe once a week. Now it's once every four days. And you say there's a bit less pain during sex. You* are *getting better . . .*

Amy generates a report at each patient visit, which typically occurs once and sometimes twice a week, but she assesses progress on a monthly basis—the same thing we recommend for your personal tracking. There are ups and downs, but the key is the steadiness of the gains over time. It means the patients are headed in a healing direction. They *are* getting better.

Both of us recognize that the changes are incremental, but as any data analyst will tell you, incremental improvement is still improvement. Even more to the point, small changes are a message: They signal that your body is ready for change, and that tells you that you are on your way to the light at the end of the tunnel.

All we can say is: Keep at it. Wherever you fit in that seven-to-twelve-year typical gap between symptom onset and diagnosis, however many of the typically four to six physicians you consulted who told you it was "in your head" or who prescribed menopause-inducing drugs or scheduled another ablation procedure, however much you've suffered in the past and whatever you've lost, you're in the right place now. Stay there. Get proper endo treatment and continue to get your body healthy and your central nervous system cool. Keep on keeping at it.

THE ENDO COMMUNITY

Is there an endometriosis *community*? Yes, and you're part of it. Whether you are one of the one in ten women who suffer from the disease, or you know or are related to and love one of those women, or perhaps, like each of us, you are a practitioner who wants to help alleviate the suffering of women with endo, then one way or another, you are affected by this disease.

If so, you can be part of the effort to bring about some of the change the endo community needs.

What in our community needs to change? For one thing, we're still part of a society that regards "women's health issues" as separate from public health issues at large. Mary Lou Ballweg of the Endometriosis Association says the "identity of the disease of endometriosis is still tied to menstruation," around which, Ballweg contends, there remain "so many taboos and stigmas." Those taboos and stigmas are a hard-to-dislodge element of the "menstrual politics" defined by Heather Guidone, endo advocate *par excellence*, who, by the way, herself underwent more than twenty surgeries for her endo between the ages of eighteen and twenty-nine, including total hysterectomy for adenomyosis and removal of the fallopian tubes and ovaries.* Menstruation is accepted as being "cripplingly painful," in Guidone's phrase, and the woman in pain is expected to endure it silently because that's what women do.

In order to make progress in the fight against endo, it is crucial for the culture at large and women in particular to know that painful periods are *not normal.* They are not "just something we have to put up with." One "cripplingly painful" week out of every four is

---

* One of Heather's surgeries was excision surgery, and despite six years of infertility, she quickly became pregnant post-excision and gave birth to a son.

not acceptable. Instead, a serious, chronic, systemic, inflammatory illness may well lurk behind that pain. This is why educating yourself about the disease is so essential. If the medical community is still decades behind where the science on the subject is, you almost need to know more than your doctor. Reading this book has been a start. In truth, what you learned in doing so makes you more of an expert on endometriosis than a lot of healthcare practitioners.

Have you watched the movie *Endo What?* produced by Shannon McCoy Cohn? It is a documentary, in which we both appear, that really tells it like it is—a good way to learn more. Shannon has also filmed a sequel, released in 2019.

Check out the websites and books noted in our Resources section (page 261).

Take a look at the relevant social media sites; listen and learn and post.

Once you have something to say, you have two weapons in your arsenal to spread awareness of and education about this disease: your voice and this book. Are your good friends, women and men, fully aware of your endo—or of the disease itself? They need to be. Do you have kids in school? Is there a nurse employed by the school? Talk to her. Give her a copy of this book when you do. Maybe it will prompt her to take a fresh look at the girls who drop into her infirmary complaining of menstrual cramps or pelvic pain. Do the young girls in your community have access to real sex education and to information about endometriosis? Does your local library carry that information? What about your local women legislators—at the municipal, county, state level? Might they benefit from reading this book?

Do you belong to a book club? Chances are it consists mostly of women. What if you make *Beating Endo* your selection when your turn rolls around; remember that where ten women come together for anything, for instance for a book club meeting, one of you is likely to have endo. Or how about inviting friends over for a screening of *Endo What?*

Then there's the medical profession—venerable and proud, highly institutionalized, and like many institutions, sometimes rather lumbering—not exactly quick on its feet. Little by little, it is beginning to entertain change, beginning to listen to the wisdom of the East and add its value to the science of the West, beginning to come out of its separate silos and look at the whole person, not just one bit of her.

We have written earlier in this book about what we call "misdiagnosis roulette"—the estimated four to six physicians in different specialties a woman with endo consults before getting the right diagnosis. It happens not because doctors gamble with patient health; they do not. On the contrary, their choice of profession—our choice of profession—is invariably fueled by a desire to do good in the world one-on-one, patient by patient. Rather, misdiagnosis roulette happens because the research on endo is insufficient and the education on endo lags so far behind the reality that doctors are left to rely on outdated studies and the treatment guidelines still based on such studies. Both of us work hard to share with colleagues what we understand about endometriosis—through grand rounds, lecturing internationally, attending conferences, even social media—and the colleagues are glad to be enriched with the up-to-date knowledge and understanding we transmit. That is also why it is a good idea to go back to the generalists who misdiagnosed you, bringing copies of your operative and pathology reports, and gently educate them. Medical education and physical therapy education as well are just beginning to understand the ways in which women and men are different and just what that implies for the ability of physicians and physical therapists to provide the right healing. Your awareness of the problem and your ability to articulate it to others can be important in advancing the understanding we all need.

INSURANCE COVERAGE AND COST

If the diagnosis process can be roulette, insurance coverage for treatment of endo can be a crapshoot. We wrote earlier about how Amy's patients getting physical therapy for pelvic floor dysfunction are not reimbursed by their insurance carrier if their condition is "painful sex" or "inability to consummate sexual intercourse" because of their pain. Despite the fact that a vital part of a woman's life—not to mention creation of a human life—is at stake, Amy says the claim for coverage is typically dismissed as "recreational" and therefore somehow frivolous—not serious enough to warrant therapy that an insurer should cover. This is an exception; most PT diagnoses are indeed covered by insurance.

And as everyone knows well, healthcare can be costly with or without insurance, meaning that there are undoubtedly many endo sufferers for whom the prospects of good treatment are limited by financial resources.

For PT providers like Amy, the issue is simply that the reimbursement available may not match the cost of providing the level of care that is her trademark—the kind of care that helps patients beat endo. Absolutely essential to the expertise her staff of therapists possesses are continuing education and nonstop mentoring. The reasons are pretty obvious: Physical therapy is a field that is changing all the time; new developments, new techniques, improvements on old techniques pour steadily out of the pipeline, and continuing education, often requiring years of study, is the only way to keep up. It is why Amy subsidizes a huge portion of that continuing education for her staff; she also supports the mentoring of staff so that the expertise gained by one staff member gets shared with the other therapists. The return on that investment is a guarantee of excellence, but it is prohibitively expensive.

The cost issue can also become prohibitive in the case of the one treatment that can actually remove endo—excision surgery. That is because of the particular insurance code that sets the reimbursement standard for doctors performing surgical treatment for endometriosis. The code, known as CPT 58662—Current Procedural Terminology 58662—like all such codes, is created by the American Medical Association, the key professional association of physicians in the United States, dedicated to promoting "the art and science of medicine and the betterment of public health." Once a particular CPT is determined by an AMA committee of experts dedicated to that purpose, AMA editorial boards reportedly review and update the code each year, theoretically with input also provided by the American College of Obstetricians and Gynecologists (ACOG), the national professional organization for ob-gyns.

The need for such codes is not in question; CPTs provide uniformity and thereby simplify the process of claiming insurance coverage for medical treatments even as they set the reimbursement amount the insurance company pays. The problem is that with CPT 58662, uniformity and simplification fly in the face of both medical reality and common sense. The code covers surgical laparoscopy via cauterization *or* excision "of lesions of the ovary, pelvic viscera, or peritoneal surface *by any method* [italics ours] . . . when no additional tissue is removed."

Simply put, that means that in the eyes of medical insurers, all endometriosis surgical procedures are equal, and they are equally reimbursed. A single ablation procedure pays the doctor who performs the procedure the same amount as a single excision procedure pays the excision surgeon. As you can well appreciate by now, this makes no sense. The two procedures are in no way equal in the training, skill, time, and effort required to perform each; Iris knows well that some surgeries may take from sunup to sunset to complete properly. She also knows they took ten years of education and training, decades of keeping up with research and with skills training, and more than a decade of experience—on-the-job training, so to speak. She brings all of this to each patient.

But in order to perform surgery at all, she has to pay malpractice insurance. Hospitals require that. In some states, it can cost upwards of a quarter of a million dollars *per year*. Add in office rent, staff, utilities, and there 58662 still stands, reimbursing her roughly $600 per case—sometimes less, sometimes more. Often, it doesn't even pay the rent.

This is the medical-economics reality that drives so many dedicated excision surgeons to become out-of-network providers. Meanwhile, ablation continues to be the default procedure for endo, despite its limitations. And so the situation is likely to remain until we can expand endometriosis research beyond Big Pharma funding and can inspire the ACOG to update its treatment guidelines to reflect reality, not "what has always been done."

There's a word for all this: wasteful. And it means that many endo patients are not getting the best care that is available to them.

Yet, despite extensive lobbying by patients and physicians, thus far nothing has budged 58662 off its perch as the catchall treatment and reimbursement standard for endometriosis. But we're not giving up the fight. This is an issue that patients and organizations like the AAGL, the American Association of Gynecologic Laparoscopists, which works to "advance minimally invasive gynecology worldwide," the Center for Endometriosis Care, and, on Facebook, Nancy's Nook and Endo Warriors have been fighting for years.

And it is very likely all part of a bigger, wider "push" to move established thinking and established institutions a step ahead— never easy. But your voice *can* help, so join up and be heard.

It can help even more powerfully if it is joined by the voices of others. In 2018, a group of women with endo gathered in Washington, D.C., for a protest at ACOG headquarters and to lobby for improved standards of care. The year before, the then-president of the organization had famously conceded that "63 percent" of ob-gyn doctors were "uncomfortable" dealing with endo and that half did not know the disease's main symptoms. The protesting women were angry that the president then proceeded to do nothing to change the situation. Little wonder that close to nine thousand endo patients signed a petition demanding greater awareness of the disease and increased attention to those afflicted with it.

Attention must indeed be paid, as the saying goes, and the Resources section of this book (page 261) lists a number of websites and organizations that we both think of as essential participants in the fight to extend awareness of this disease afflicting one in ten women on earth. We urge you to get involved. The status quo is simply not acceptable; it must be changed, and that takes a movement. So once you have been diagnosed with endo, talk about it. Tell people. Tell your friends, tell your family. Post about it on social media.

We know: It's the last thing you feel like doing when you are sick yourself, when the pain and discomfort and sheer unfairness of your disease have you feeling down and out. But did anything important ever happen without people making it happen? And, as the saying goes: If not now, when? And if not you, who?

Well, one answer to that question is: us. We're there with you. When we think back on the time when we first connected our minds and our practices, it felt like we were two lonely pioneers setting out on an unmarked trail where we saw very, very few other travelers. That has begun to change—not yet dramatically, but noticeably.

Iris recalls how in the years following her fellowship, she set herself to perfect her skills as an excision surgeon because that particular expertise, she felt, was all she had to offer her patients. Then came that study on post-op excision patients confirming what Iris's own experience was showing her—namely, that even *with* the surgery, patients did not get 100 percent better—and it prompted her quest to figure out why. The quest took her into other fields of medicine, to ancient medical practices from distant cultures, and beyond the "walls" of medicine itself into the mind-body connection. What she learned sparked an evolution in her very practice and shaped the multimodal, integrated palette of healing she is able to offer today to patients—from teenagers with endo to women of all ages suffering chronic pain.

For her part, Amy had noted the same inability of standard medical practice to meet the needs of a great number of the patients she treated. As with Iris, the relief Amy was able to provide was palpable, and she was grateful to be able to deliver it, but it was clear that these patients were up against something that PT alone, like excision surgery alone, could not overcome. Her revelation came at that 2005 conference in Sydney, Australia, when only a tiny minority of the expert medical and PT practitioners in the audience could identify endo in the photographs. Again, just as with Iris, the revelation spurred her to explore more deeply what she was up against, but she wasn't really sure where to go next, either; the path was in no way straightforward—until she made the connection with a small number of like-minded practitioners committed to treating endo.

This book marks how far we have come and where we are now. Each of us is still a bit of an anomaly in our individual professions, but we both remain committed to helping women reclaim the lives that this disease has stolen from them. The trail we embarked on years ago is still a bit lonely, but it has a few more travelers today than it did then, and there seem to be more signposts as well. We can hear the organizations working to spread awareness of endo raise their voices more and more clearly with every passing day. We hope this book will help spread the word as well.

And the word is this: You *can* beat endo, and you are not fighting alone.

ACKNOWLEDGMENTS

You might think it would be difficult for two separate individuals who are coauthoring a book to determine whose help to acknowledge *first*. But for us, there was no contest: Our patients have been our inspiration and our purpose. Our desire to help them regain their lives and live them to the fullest is what has impelled us to write this book.

Key helpers in the task are all the contributors—the expert doctors, PTs, nutritionists, psychologists, non-opioid-pushing pain docs—who share our passion and who gave of their time and expertise to help us explain the many varied aspects of endometriosis and to dig deeper into the issues it raises. It takes a village of very astute, dedicated professionals to write a book like this, and we are grateful for the contributions of all "our" villagers.

For getting the book off the ground, we thank our agent, Sarah-Jane Freymann, and for helping to get the book out of us and into a manuscript, we thank Susanna Margolis. At HarperCollins, we are grateful for the support and help of our team of editors, Julie Will and Haley Swanson, of copyeditor Leda Scheintaub, and of the entire production team and marketing squad Laura Cole, Emily VanDerwerken, Milan Bozic, and Leah Carlson-Stanisic.

We also want to acknowledge three veteran Endo Warriors who have been essential to us both over the years and have also gifted us with their friendship. Mary Lou Ballweg, Heather Guidone, and

Nancy Petersen have been overflowing fountains of information and advice in phone calls, meetings, conferences, and messages. Iris calls Heather her "all-things-endo lifeline," cherishes the annual wisdom delivered by Mary Lou at AAGL conferences and in phone calls over the years, and regards Nancy as the exemplar of tireless dedication to the fight against endo. To both of us, they are the undisputed and irrepressible doyennes of endo awareness, and this book would not have been possible without them.

But in addition to our collective thanks, each of us has some individual acknowledgments to make:

IRIS

I cannot express too often or too strongly my gratitude to my mentors, Dr. Harry Reich and Dr. C. Y. Liu, for sharing their passion with me.

I want to thank my parents—not just for our family life but for the special gifts each gave that I now try to exhibit to my own children. My father, Dr. Nicholas Kerin, has been my role model— dedicated to his patients, author of nearly a hundred articles and chapters, and always available to give me spot-on advice as both a dad and a medical professional. He persistently—relentlessly!— encouraged me to pursue the dream of writing this book, not to put it off, to keep at it. Look, Dad, it's done. My mother, Jeny Kerin, not only created the warm home I grew up in but still leaves me after every visit well fed, well rested, and well loved.

Above all, I want to thank my family for their patience over these last two years as I chased the dream of this book—my daughters, Alexandra and Olivia, and my husband, Larry. I am particularly grateful for the guidance my husband offered, for encouraging me to bounce endless ideas off him, and for exemplifying unconditional love while sharing with me our joint devotion towards women with endo.

AMY

I am grateful to all my many pelvic health mentors, especially the International Pelvic Pain Society, who have been educating me in endometriosis treatment for nearly two decades. I began to understand how much I learned from them when I realized I had become a pelvic health mentor myself.

I also want to thank mentors in a broader sense—my parents—for their unconditional love, support, and for always pushing me to be the best I could be. Thanks as well to my extended family—for as many reasons as there are family members.

I am grateful also to the entire Beyond Basics PT staff—another extended family—for their patience and for putting up with the sudden stops and starts and occasional chaos that writing this book has imposed.

Above all, I am grateful to my own family—my husband, Travis Wood, and my children, Zachary and Zoe Wood, for their patience, their endless support, and their love. And a special shout-out to the inimitable Sonia François, babysitter *par excellence*. Without all of them, this book really could not have been written.

RESOURCES

Information, Treatment, Support, Advocacy

Amy Stein, DPT
www.beyondbasicsphysicaltherapy.com
www.healpelvicpain.com
Facebook, Instagram, Twitter: beyondbasicspt
(212) 354-2622

Iris Kerin Orbuch, MD
www.lagyndr.com
www.nycrobotic.com
Instagram: dririsorbuch
(310) 850-0051

ENDOMETRIOSIS

Thankfully, there are literally thousands of websites and social media groups and organizations dedicated to endometriosis. Here are some of those we have mentioned in this book.

Social Media: Nancy's Nook Endometriosis Education, Endo
     Warriors

Endometriosis Association: www.endometriosisassn.org

EndoWhat?: www.endowhat.com

Casey Berna: www.caseyberna.com

Endopaedia: www.endopaedia.info

Endometriosis Research Center: www.endocenter.org

AAGL: www.aagl.org

Center for Endometriosis Care: www.centerforendo.com

The Endometriosis Coalition: Instagram: @theendo.co; contact:
     Jenneh@theendo.co

Endometriosis Summit: https://www.theendometriosissummit.com;
     Facebook: The Endometriosis Summit; Instagram: @endometrio
     sissummit

Pelvic Health Summit: https://www.pelvichealthsummit.com; In-
     stagram: @pelvichealthsummit

EndoInvisible: www.endoinvisible.org

Extrapelvic Not Rare: www.extrapelvicnotrare.org

Endometriosis & Me: Facebook: Endometriosis and me

Endometriosis Australia: https://www.endometriosisaustralia
     .org

Endometriosis.org

Endometriosis New Zealand: https://nzendo.org.nz/

PT

Blogs: beyondbasicspt.com/blog; blogtalkradio.com/pelvicmessenger

American Physical Therapy Association: www.apta.org

Herman & Wallace Pelvic Rehabilitation: www.hermanwallace
     .com

NUTRITION

Environmental Working Group: www.ewg.org
www.womensvoices.org
www.nourishingmeals.com
www.integrativewomenshealthinstitute.com
Institute for Functional Medicine: www.ifm.org
www.thrivemarket.com

ENVIRONMENT

Environmental Working Group: www.ewg.org
www.badgerbalm.com
www.credobeauty.com
www.rmsbeauty.com
www.thedetoxmarket.com
www.paiskincare.us
www.beautycounter.com
www.madesafe.org
www.savvywomensalliance.org

MINDFULNESS

www.calm.com
www.headspace.com
www.buddhify.com
www.lumosity.com
www.breethe.com
CD/App: *Guided Meditation for Mindfulness Living* by Alexandra
   Milspaw www.4directionscounseling.com

Recognise apps from the NOI Group, available on iTunes or Google
  Store

Dr. Alex Milspaw's YouTube channel for meditations at https://
  www.youtube.com/channel/UCeGEr6hWrTjh-SZxKzwPJDg
  and her website at www.4dcounseling.com

SEX

Recommended products for dyspareunia and deep penetrative pain:

Ohnut: www.ohnut.co; hello@ohnut.co

Organic coconut oil (incompatible with latex condoms)

Organic olive oil (incompatible with latex condoms)

Yes lubricant: www.yesyesyes.org (not condom-compatible)

Good Clean Love (condom-compatible options): www.goodclean
  love.com; service@goodcleanlove.com

OTHER

Interstitial Cystitis Association: www.ichelp.org

Interstitial Cystitis Network: www.ic-network.org

International Pelvic Pain Society: www.pelvicpain.org

American Fibromyalgia Syndrome Association: www.afsafund
  .org

American Urological Association: www.auanet.org; (410) 727-1100

Chronic Fatigue and Immune Dysfunction Syndrome: www.cfids
  .org

International Foundation for Gastrointestinal Disorders: www
  .iffgd.org

International Society for the Study of Vulvovaginal Disease (ISSVD):
  www.issvd.org

International Society for the Study of Women's Sexual Health:
www.isswsh.org

International Urogynecological Association: www.iuga.org

National Vulvodynia Association: www.nva.org

Pudendal Neuralgia Association: www.pudendalassociation.org

PELVIC PAIN

Products, Supplies

Video: *Healing Pelvic and Abdominal Pain Featuring Amy Stein*—
available as DVD or digital download: www.healpelvicpain.com

Dilators and wands: www.icrelief.com, www.soulsource.com

Other Pelvic Pain Resources

www.pelvicpainsolutions.com

www.cmtmedical.com

Cushions

www.cushionyourassets.com

BOOKS

Endometriosis

Ballweg, Mary Lou. *Endometriosis: The Complete Reference for Taking Charge of Your Health.*

Ballweg, Mary Lou. *The Endometriosis Sourcebook.*

Bowick, Samantha. *Living with Endometriosis.*

Evans, Dr. Susan. *Endometriosis and Pelvic Pain.*

Mills, Dian Shepperson, and Michael Vernon. *Endometriosis: A Key to Healing Through Nutrition.*

Redwine, Dr. David. *100 Questions & Answers About Endometriosis.*

Physical Therapy

Stein, Amy. *Heal Pelvic Pain.* McGraw Hill, 2008.

Jeffcoat, Heather, DPT. *Sex Without Pain.* Active Orange Publishing, 2014.

Prendergast, Stephanie A., and Elizabeth H. Akincilar. *Pelvic Pain Explained: What You Need to Know.* Rowman & Littlefield Publishers, 2017.

Nutrition

Drummond, Jessica. *Nutrition for Relieving Pelvic Pain: Fueling the Patient/Practitioner Healing Partnership.*

Other

Butler, David, and G. Lorimer Moseley. *Explain Pain.* NOI Group, 2014.

Coady, Deborah, and Nancy Fish. *Healing Painful Sex: A Woman's Guide to Confronting, Diagnosing, and Treating Sexual Pain.* Seal Press, 2011.

Goldstein, Andrew, MD, and Marianne Brandon, PhD. *Reclaiming Desire: 4 Keys to Finding Your Lost Libido.*

Goldstein, Andrew, Caroline Pukall, and Irwin Goldstein. *When Sex Hurts: A Woman's Guide to Banishing Sexual Pain.* Da Capo Lifelong Books, 2011.

NOTES

1. David B. Redwine, MD, "Conservative laparoscopic excision of endometriosis by sharp dissection: life table analysis of reoperation and persistent or recurrent disease," *Fertility and Sterility*, vol. 56, no. 4 (October 1991).

2. Tom Gellhaus, "It's Time We Talk About Endometriosis," *The President's Blog, ACOG*, March 21, 2017, acogpresident.org /?p=1443

3. P. Signorile, et al., "Embryologic Origin of Endometriosis: Analysis of 101 Human Female Fetuses," *J. Cell. Physiol.* vol. 227 (2012): 1653–56.

4. Private communication via email to Iris Orbuch, November 17, 2018.

5. Endometriosis Association. 2018. "Research and Translational Medicine for Endometriosis." https://endometriosisassn.org /our-work/endometriosisresearch

6. Dr. Hazama is also vice-chair of the scientific education committee of the International Pelvic Pain Society.

7. Based, with gratitude, on the groundbreaking work of Travell, Simons, and Simons, articulated in a seminal work in two volumes: D. G. Simons, J. G. Travell, and L. S. Simons, *Myofascial Pain and Dysfunction: The Trigger Point Manual*, Baltimore: Williams & Wilkins, 1983, Vol. 2, 1992.

8. J. M. Weiss, "Pelvic floor myofascial trigger points: manual

therapy for interstitial cystitis and the urgency-frequency syndrome," *J. Urol.* vol. 166, no. 6 (2001): 2226–31.

9.   PNF is a philosophy and a concept of treatment developed in the 1940s by Dr. Herman Kabat and taught by Margaret Knott. See *PNF in Practice: An Illustrated Guide*, third edition, by Susan Adler, Dominiek Beckers, and Math Buck (Springer, 2008).

10.   Maurice K. Chung, et al., "The Evil Twins of Chronic Pelvic Pain Syndrome: Endometriosis and Interstitial Cystitis," *JSLS*, vol. 6, no. 4 (Oct–Dec 2002): 311–14.

11.   P. Maroun, et al., "Relevance of gastrointestinal symptoms in endometriosis," *Australian and New Zealand Journal of Obstetrics and Gynecology*, vol. 49 (2009): 411–14.

12.   I. Kerin Orbuch, et al., "Laparoscopic treatment of recurrent small bowel obstruction secondary to ileal endometriosis," *Journal of Minimally Invasive Gynecology*, vol. 14, no. 1 (2006): 113–15.

13.   Dr. Goldstein is the director of the Centers for Vulvovaginal Disorders in Washington, D.C. and New York City and is a past president of the International Society for the Study of Women's Sexual Health (ISSWSH), and is currently a Clinical Professor at the George Washington University School of Medicine.

14.   Herman & Wallace Inc., second edition (2010): New York, HermanWallace.com.

15.   Cofounder of the Pelvic Health and Rehabilitation Center and one-time head of the International Pelvic Pain Society. Coauthor, with Elizabeth H. Akincilar, of *Pelvic Pain Explained: What You Need to Know* (Rowman & Littlefield Publishers, 2017).

16.   Sandra Hilton, et al., "The Puzzle of Pelvic Pain—A Reha-

bilitation Framework for Balancing Tissue Dysfunction and Central Sensitization, I: Pain Physiology and Evaluation for the Physical Therapist," *Journal of Women's Health Physical Therapy*, vol. 35, no. 3 (September/December 2011).

17. A. Levesque, T. Riant, S. Ploteau, et al., "Clinical Criteria of Central Sensitization in Chronic Pelvic and Perineal Pain (Convergence PP Criteria): Elaboration of a Clinical Evaluation Tool Based on Formal Expert Consensus," *Pain Med.*, vol. 19, no. 10 (2018): 2009–2015.

18. Melissa M. Smarr, et al., "Endocrine disrupting chemicals and endometriosis," *Fertility and Sterility*, vol. 106, no. 4 (2016).

19. Melissa M. Smarr, et al., "Endocrine disrupting chemicals and endometriosis," *Fertility and Sterility*, vol. 106, no. 4 (2016).

20. A. Doll, et al., "Mindful attention to breath regulates emotions via increased amygdala-prefrontal cortex connectivity," *NeuroImage*, vol. 134 (2016): 305–13.

21. Ibid.

22. Katha Upanishad 2.6.10–11.

23. J. Wright, et al., "A randomized trial of excision versus ablation for mild endometriosis," *Fertility and Sterility*, vol. 83, no. 6 (June 2005), copyright © 2005 American Society for Reproductive Medicine, published by Elsevier Inc. doi:10.1016/j.fertnstert.2004.11.066.

24. Martin Healey, et al., "To Excise or Ablate Endometriosis? A Prospective, Randomized, Double-Blinded Trial After 5-Year Follow-Up," *Journal of Minimally Invasive Gynecology*, vol. 21 (2014): 999–1004.

25. J. Pundir, MD, et al., "Laparoscopic Excision Versus Ablation for Endometriosis-Associated Pain: An Updated Systematic Review and Meta-analysis," *Journal of Minimally Invasive Gynecology*, vol. 24, no. 5 (July/August 2017).

26. E. Saridogan, "Endometriosis in Teenagers," *Women's Health*, vol. 11, no. 5 (2005): 705–09.

27. T. Dowlut-McElroy, et al., "Endometriosis in Adolescents," www.co-obgyn.com, vol. 29, no. 5 (October 2017).

28. E. Saridogan, "Endometriosis in Teenagers," *Women's Health*, vol. 11, no. 5 (2005): 705–09.

29. E. Dun, et al., *JSLS*, vol. 19, no. 2 (April–June 2015).

30. M. L. Ballweg, "Big picture of endometriosis helps provide guidance on approach to teens: comparative historical data show endo starting younger, is more severe," J. Pediatr. Adolesc. Gynecol. 16 (3 Suppl) (2003): S21–26.

31. C. A. Smith, et al., "Acupuncture performed around the time of embryo transfer: a systematic review and meta-analysis," *Reprod. Biomed. Online*, Jan 2, 2019, doi: 10.1016/j.rbmo.2018.12.038. (Epub ahead of print.) Review. C. A. Smith, et. al., "The effects of acupuncture on the secondary outcomes of anxiety and quality of life for women undergoing IVF: A randomized controlled trial," *Acta. Obstet. Gynecol. Scand.*, Dec. 28, 2018, doi: 10.1111/aogs.13528. (Epub ahead of print.)

INDEX

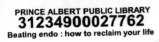